Avoiding Errors in
Paediatrics

To Elaine, Katie and Ben
Rachel and Anna
and Anne

Avoiding Errors in
Paediatrics

Joseph E. Raine

MD, FRCPCH, DCH
Consultant Paediatrician
Whittington Hospital
London, UK

Kate Williams

MA (Oxon)
Partner
Radcliffes LeBrasseur Solicitors
Leeds, UK

Jonathan Bonser

BA (Oxon)
Consultant in the Healthcare Department of
Fishburns LLP, Solicitors
London, UK
Former Head of the Claims and Legal Services
Department of the Leeds office of the Medical Protection Society

WILEY-BLACKWELL

A John Wiley & Sons, Ltd., Publication

This edition first published 2013 © 2013 by John Wiley & Sons, Ltd.

Wiley-Blackwell is an imprint of John Wiley & Sons, formed by the merger of Wiley's global Scientific, Technical and Medical business with Blackwell Publishing.

Registered office: John Wiley & Sons, Ltd, The Atrium, Southern Gate, Chichester, West Sussex, PO19 8SQ, UK

Editorial offices: 9600 Garsington Road, Oxford, OX4 2DQ, UK
The Atrium, Southern Gate, Chichester, West Sussex, PO19 8SQ, UK
111 River Street, Hoboken, NJ 07030-5774, USA

For details of our global editorial offices, for customer services and for information about how to apply for permission to reuse the copyright material in this book please see our website at www.wiley.com/wiley-blackwell.

Library of Congress Cataloging-in-Publication Data

Raine, Joseph E.
   Avoiding errors in paediatrics / Joseph E. Raine, Kate Williams, Jonathan Bonser.
      p. ; cm.
   Includes bibliographical references and index.
   ISBN 978-0-470-65868-0 (pbk. : alk. paper) – ISBN 978-1-118-44193-0 (eMobi) –
   ISBN 978-1-118-44194-7 (ePDF/ebook) – ISBN 978-1-118-44195-4 (epub)
   I. Williams, Kate, MA. II. Bonser, Jonathan. III. Title.
   [DNLM: 1. Medical Errors–prevention & control–Case Reports.   2. Pediatrics–legislation & jurisprudence–Case Reports.   3. Medical Errors–legislation & jurisprudence–Case Reports.
4. Pediatrics–ethics–Case Reports.   WS 100]
   610.28′9–dc23

                                                                                 2012024676

A catalogue record for this book is available from the British Library.

Cover design: Sarah Dickinson

Set in 10.5/13 pt Minion by Aptara® Inc., New Delhi, India
Printed and bound in Malaysia by Vivar Printing Sdn Bhd

1   2013

Contents

Part 3 Investigating and dealing with errors

Contributors

Giles Armstrong
Consultant Paediatrician
Whittington Hospital
London
Part 1, Section 1: Failure to Identify a Sick Child, Failures in Resuscitation
Cases: 4, 29, 32, 36

Edward Broadhurst
Formerly Consultant Neonatologist
Whittington Hospital
London
Part 1, Section 1: Inability to Perform Practical Procedures Competently
Cases: 10, 13, 14, 18, 24

Aubrey Cunnington
Specialist Registrar in Paediatric Infectious Diseases and Immunology
Great Ormond Street Hospital
London
Cases: 12, 16, 26-28, 34

Joanne Haswell
Barrister; Director, InPractice Training
London
Part 3: The Role of Hospital Staff, External Investigators, Hospital Investigations, The Role of the Doctor

Alistair Hewitt
Partner, Radcliffes LeBrasseur
Leeds
Part 3: Coroner's Court, Criminal Matters

Kate Hill
Solicitor, Radcliffes LeBrasseur
Managing Director, InPractice Training,
London
Part 3: The Role of Hospital Staff, External Investigators, Hospital Investigations, The Role of the Doctor

Sasha Howard
Paediatric Clinical Fellow
Royal London Hospital
London
Case 19

Heather Mackinnon
Consultant Paediatrician
Whittington Hospital
London
Part 1, Section 1: Sources of Error in Child Protection
Cases: 6, 23, 33

Gopa Sen
Locum Consultant Paediatrician
Whittington Hospital
London
Case 8
Section 3: How Hospitals Try to Prevent Errors and Their Recurrence

Joanna Walker
Consultant Paediatrician
Portsmouth Hospital NHS Trust
Portsmouth
Cases: 11, 15, 17, 25, 30, 31,

Acknowledgements

The authors would like to thank Dr Nick Owen, Consultant Radiologist, Whittington Hospital; Dr Tony Wheeler, Consultant Community Paediatrician, Whittington Hospital; and Dianna Scarrott, Head of Information and Knowledge Management, National Clinical Assessment Service, National Patient Safety Agency for their help and advice with different sections of the book.

Foreword

Sometimes we may learn more from a man's errors, than from his virtues.
—*Henry Wadsworth Longfellow*

Paediatrics is an exciting, rewarding and diverse speciality. Doctors who opt for a career in paediatrics know that the high intensity, challenging aspects of the work are balanced in equal measure by the satisfaction of supporting children and families through both acute and long-term illness. However, every practising clinician lives with the uncomfortable truth that the practice of medicine is an error-prone business; and if the stakes are high in all specialities, they are even more so in the care of children.

It goes without saying that no doctor or nurse leaves home in the morning with the intention of harming a child. Indeed, we can only function in the workplace by putting to the furthest recesses of our mind the notion that our actions, in the worst-case scenario, could result in a child's death. Nonetheless, the guilt and self-recrimination that follow even the most trivial of errors are emotions that every clinician would wish to avoid. And that is the great appeal of this book. It is not an academic treatise on the extensive literature about error, human factors, system failure and organizational accidents. Because the busiest, most hard-pressed paediatrician – arguably at greatest risk of making an error – is the one least likely to read such a book. Rather this is an accessible and engaging book, written in a way that will draw its readers in through the appeal of case studies.

For those who do want a helicopter overview of the key causes of errors and the legal context, that is provided in a short punchy style in the first section of the book. The systematic reader will start there first, whilst those who take more of a 'bumble-bee' approach to flitting around books will fly straight to the cases studies. These cannot be read passively! They are devised so as to challenge as well as inform, forcing the reader to really think through what they would have done in the circumstances, before presenting the expert opinion and legal comment, and rounding up with key learning points. Each one can be read in a few minutes at a bus stop or in a lull between patients in a clinic – and any one could make the difference between a clinician making or averting the same mistake. The final section wraps up with a practical account of investigation and management of errors and their fallout.

Every serious paediatric error is a tragedy for the child and family involved. Perhaps the greatest tragedy of all, as set out at the beginning of this book, is that errors fall into recurrent themes that are repeated by successive generations of doctors. Families of children who have suffered from a medical error frequently say that they don't want the same thing to ever happen to another child. This book is the most effective way to widely share learning from the case studies, and in doing so to give something back – albeit anonymously – to the children and families involved. If each case described stops even one similar recurrence it will be a worthwhile outcome.

Hilary Cass
President, Royal College of Paediatrics and Child Health

Abbreviations

ACRM	Anaesthesia Crisis Resource Management
ALL	acute lymphoblastic leukaemia
ALP	alkaline phosphatase
ALSG	Advanced Life Support Group
ALT	alanine transaminase
APLS	Advanced Paediatric Life Support
ARDS	Adult Respiratory Distress Syndrome
AXR	abdominal X-ray
BP	blood pressure
CDOP	The Child Death Overview Panel
CP	child protection
CPAP	continuous positive airways pressure
CPD	continuous professional development
CPS	Crown Prosecution Service
CRP	c reactive protein
CRT	capillary refill time
CSC	Children's Social Care
CSF	cerebrospinal fluid
CT	computerised tomography scan
CXR	chest X-ray
DAT	direct agglutination test
DGH	district general hospital
DKA	diabetic ketoacidosis
ECG	electrocardiogram
ED	emergency department
EEG	electroencephalogram
ESBL	extended spectrum beta-lactamase
ESR	erythrocyte sedimentation rate
FBC	full blood count
FY1 and 2	foundation year 1 and 2 doctors (most junior doctor training grades)
GBS	Group B streptococcal
GCS	Glasgow Coma Score
GMC	General Medical Council
GP	general practitioner
Hb	haemoglobin
HDU	high dependency unit
HIV	human immunodeficiency virus
HQIP	Healthcare Quality Improvement Partnership
HV	heath visitor
IPPV	intermittent positive pressure ventilation
IT	intrathecal
IV	intravenous
LFTs	liver function tests
LP	lumbar puncture
LSCB	Local Safeguarding Children Board
MDDUS	Medical and Dental Defence Union of Scotland
MDO	Medical Defence Organisation
MDU	Medical Defence Union
Mg	magnesium
MHPS	Maintaining High Professional Standards in the Modern NHS
MPS	Medical Protection Society
MRI	magnetic resonance imaging
MRSA	Methicillin Resistant Staphylococcus aureus
NCAS	National Clinical Assessment Service
NHS	National Health Service
NHSLA	National Health Service Litigation Authority
NICE	National Institute for Clinical Excellence
NICU	neonatal intensive care unit
PALS	paediatric advanced life support
PALS	Patient Advice and Liaison Service
PCR	polymerase chain reaction
PET	Paediatric Epilepsy Training
PEW	Paediatric Early Warning
PHHI	persistent hyperinsulinaemic hypoglycaemia of infancy
PICU	paediatric intensive care unit
PM	postmortem
POC	Paediatric Oncology Centre
POSCU	Paediatric Oncology Shared Care Unit
PVL-SA	Panton-Valentine Leukocidin producing *S. aureus*

RCPCH	Royal College of Paediatrics and Child Health	**TPHA**	Treponema pallidum particle agglutination assay
SaO2	oxygen saturation	**TPO**	thyroid peroxidase antibody
SPOC	single point of contact	**TSH**	thyroid stimulating hormone
ST 1-8	specialist training grades 1–8; grades 1–3 are equivalent to senior house officer standard and grades 4-8 to registrar standard	**TSS**	toxic shock syndrome
		U and E's	urea and electrolytes
		US	ultrasound
		WBC	white blood cells
SUFE	slipped upper femoral epiphysis	**WCC**	white cell count
TFT	thyroid function tests	**ZIG**	zoster immune globulin

Introduction

In 2000, a committee established by the Department of Health, chaired by the then Chief Medical Officer, Professor Liam Donaldson, published its report *An Organisation with a Memory*. The report recognized that the vast majority of NHS care was of a very high clinical standard and that serious failures were uncommon given the volume of care provided. However, when failures do occur their consequences can be devastating for the individual patients and their families. The health care workers feel guilt and distress. Like a ripple effect, the mistakes also undermine the public's confidence in the Health Service. Last, but not least, these adverse events have a huge cumulative financial effect. Updating the figures provided in the report, in 2010/11, the NHS Litigation Authority (the NHSLA is the body that handles negligence claims against NHS Trusts in England) paid out £863,400,000 for medical negligence claims (these figures take no account of the costs incurred by the Medical Defence Organisations for General Practice and private health care). The report commented ruefully that often these failures have a familiar ring to them; many could be avoided 'if only the lessons of experience were properly learned'.

The Committee writing the report also noted that there is a vast reservoir of clinical data from negligence claims that remains untapped. They were gently critical of the Health Service as being par excellence a passive learning organization; like a school teacher writing an end of term report, they classified the NHS a poor learner – could do better. On a more positive note, the report stated that 'There is significant potential to extract valuable learning by focusing, specialty by specialty, on the main areas of practice that have resulted in litigation.' It acknowledged that learning from adverse clinical events is a key component of clinical governance and is an important component in delivering the Government's quality agenda for the NHS.

The NHSLA has reported that its present (as of 2011) estimate for all potential liabilities, existing and expected claims, is £16.8 billion. At the time *An Organisation with a Memory* was written, this figure stood at £2.4 billion. (These sums are actuarially calculated figures that are based on both known and as yet unknown claims, some of which may not surface for many years to come. They should not be confused with the figure of £863,000,000 mentioned above, which was the sum actually paid out in one year.) The NHSLA also reported that the number of negligence claims rose from 6652 in 2009/10 to 8655 in 2010/11. While the increases in these figures may be due to the increased readiness of patients to pursue negligence claims and the very significant costs of claims inflation, rather than any marked decline in the standard of care provided by the NHS, the statistics clearly show that there is still room for improvement in the care provided to patients. It is this gap in the standard of care that we, the authors, wish to address through this book.

An Organisation with a Memory as a report tried to take a fresh look at the nature of mistakes within the NHS. It looked at fields of activity outside health care, such as the airline industry. The committee commented that there were two ways of viewing human error: the person-centred approach and the systems approach. The person-centred approach focuses on the individual, his inattention, forgetfulness and carelessness. Its correctives are aimed at individuals and propagate a blame culture. The systems approach, on the other hand, takes a holistic view of the reasons for failure. It recognizes that many of the problems facing large organizations are complex and result from the interplay of many factors: errors often arise from the cumulative effect of a number of small mistakes; they cannot always be pinned on one blameworthy individual. This approach starts from the position that humans do make mistakes and that errors are inevitable, but tries to change the environment in which people work, so that fewer mistakes will be made.

The systems approach does not, however, absolve individuals of their responsibilities. Rather, it suggests that we should not automatically assume that we should look for an individual to blame for an adverse outcome. The authors of *An Organisation with a Memory* acknowledged that clinical practice did differ from many hi-tech industries. The airline industry, for example, can place a number of hi-tech safeguards between danger and harm. This is often not possible in many fields of clinical practice, where the human elements are often the last and the most important defences. 'In surgery,' they wrote, 'very little lies between the scalpel and some untargeted nerve or blood vessel other than the skill and training of the surgeon.' We believe that this difference is key to understanding the nature of error in healthcare and why we have placed such great emphasis on case studies that show how doctors make mistakes in treating their patients.

The committee felt that the NHS had for too long taken a person-centred approach to the errors made by its employees and that this had stifled improvement. They called for a change in the culture of the NHS and a move away from what they saw as its blame culture. More than a decade has passed since the writing of the report and there has been little change in attitudes. A sea change is required. We want to see an NHS that promotes a safety culture, rather than a blame culture, a culture where there are multiple safeguards built into the system.

However, the legal system in which the medical services operate does not foster such an approach. Although coroners can now comment on the strengths and weaknesses of systems in the form of narrative verdicts, in general, the medical complaints and litigation process still tends to focus on the actions of individuals rather than the failings of the system. Perhaps the most glaring example of this person-centred approach can be seen in the way the General Medical Council treats medical practitioners, when they receive a complaint. In that forum, doctors are expected to meet personal professional standards and will be held to account if they fall short of them in any way. Yet they may find themselves working in an environment that at times seems to conflict with those professional standards.

As authors, we believe that the committee of *An Organisation with a Memory* were right, when they wrote that many useful lessons can be learnt from the bitter experience of errors and litigation and that this can best be done by looking specialty by specialty at those areas of practice where errors are most frequently made. Thus, we have produced a book looking at paediatric errors. It is to be the first of a series of such books, each concentrating on a separate specialty.

If doctors are to learn lessons from their errors and litigation, then they must have some understanding of the underlying processes. Thus, in Part 1, Section 1 (Errors and their causes), we discuss types of medical error, both person-centred and systems errors. We have also summarised our research into the commonest errors in paediatrics, their types and outcomes. In Part 1, Section 2 (Medico-legal aspects), we cover the basic legal concepts relevant to medical care: negligence, consent and confidentiality.

The heart of the book is Part 2. Here, we set out a number of case studies on common mistakes in paediatrics. Each case is drawn from real scenarios, anonymised to protect patient confidentiality and is supplemented with legal comment. Most cases concern failures to diagnose an illness, the commonest source of error in medical treatment. In Part 1, we have at various points cross-referred to relevant cases in Part 2.

Finally, Part 3 provides a practical guide to the various forms of complaint that a doctor may encounter, how they may affect him and what he can do to protect his interests.

Our aim is to provide a book that will go some way to meet the challenges laid down at the turn of the millennium in *An Organisation with a Memory*. We hope that it will reduce the number of clinical errors and improve the standard of care provided by individual paediatricians and Paediatric Departments throughout the country.

References and further reading

Department of Health (2000) An Organisation with a Memory, the report of an expert group on learning from adverse events in the NHS, chaired by the Chief Medical Officer. http://www.dh.gov.uk/en/ Publicationsandstatistics/Publications/PublicationsPolicyAndGuidance/ Browsable/DH_4098184

National Health Service Litigation Authority (2011) The National Health Service Litigation Authority Report and Accounts 2010-11. http://www. nhsla.com/NR/rdonlyres/3F5DFA84-2463-468B-890C-42C0FC16D4D6/ 0/NHSLAAnnualReportandAccounts2011.pdf

Section 1: Errors and their causes

A few words about error

If our aim is to reduce the number of clinical errors, then we must explain what we mean by 'error'. The Oxford English Dictionary defines 'an error' as a mistake. This is self-evident and does not really help us, the authors, to define our goal.

We could define our aim by looking at the end-result of errors and say that we want to prevent poor patient outcomes. That must be our primary concern, but our aim is broader; many mistakes can be rectified before any serious harm is done.

We could look at the seriousness of the error, how 'bad' the mistake actually was. Some errors could be so crass and the consequences so serious that they can be labelled 'criminal' by one and all and in fact some cases are investigated by the police and come before the criminal courts, as we shall see later. Other errors are the sort that only become obvious with the benefit of hindsight and could be made by anyone, even the best of doctors. In short, we want to look at all errors across the spectrum. What we hope to achieve is to raise the standard of care provided to patients, so that mistakes of all kinds are reduced.

Learning from system failures – the vincristine case

The way that the courts look at error is to focus on the acts of individuals and to ascribe fault to particular doctors, if their treatment of the patient falls below the standard of the *Bolam* test (see Part 1, Section 2, below). But as mentioned in our Introduction, there is another way of looking at errors and that is to consider system failures.

In order to illustrate the difference between system failures and individual fault, the authors of *An Organisation with a Memory* examined a case concerning the maladministration of the drug vincristine. The mistake cost the patient, a child, his life. A number of shortcomings occurred during the child's stay in the hospital. We believe that it would be useful to set out what happened in the lead up to this child's death, pointing out at each stage the failings that occurred. We will then provide a more detailed discussion of the general lessons that can be learnt from the case.

The following is taken with minor amendment from *An Organisation with a Memory*. It is a classic example of how a number of small mistakes can add

Avoiding Errors in Paediatrics, First Edition. Joseph E. Raine, Kate Williams and Jonathan Bonser.
© 2013 John Wiley & Sons, Ltd. Published 2013 by Blackwell Publishing Ltd.

up to a massive error and end with a fatality. The comments in italics provide a brief analysis of the faults that occurred:

A child was being treated in a district general hospital (DGH). He was due to receive chemotherapy under a general anaesthetic at a specialist centre. He should have been fasted for 6 hours prior to the anaesthetic, but was allowed to eat and drink before leaving the DGH.

Fasting error. Poor communication between the DGH and the specialist centre.

When he arrived at the specialist centre, there were no beds available on the oncology ward, so he was admitted to a mixed-specialty 'outlier' ward.

Lack of organizational resources; there were no beds available for specialized treatment. The patient was placed in an environment where the staff had no specialist oncology expertise.

The patient's notes were lost and were not available to the ward staff on admission.

Loss of patient information.

The patient was due to receive intravenous vincristine, to be administered by a specialist oncology nurse on the ward, and intrathecal (spinal) methotrexate, to be administered in the operating theatre by an oncology Specialist Registrar. No oncology nurse specialist was available on the ward.

Communication failure between the oncology department and the outlier ward. Absence of policy and resources to deal with the demands placed on the system by outlier wards, including shortage of specialist staff.

Vincristine and methotrexate were transported together to the ward by a housekeeper instead of being kept separate at all times.

Drug delivery error due to noncompliance with hospital policy, which was that the drugs must be kept separate at all times. Communication error: the outlier ward was not aware of this policy.

The housekeeper who took the drugs to the ward informed staff that both drugs were to go to theatre with the patient.

Communication error. Incorrect information communicated. Poor delivery practice, allowing drugs to be delivered to outlier wards by inexperienced staff.

The patient was consented by a junior doctor. He was consented only for intrathecal (IT) methotrexate and not for intravenous vincristine.

Poor consenting practice. Junior doctor allowed to take consent. Consenting error.

A junior doctor abbreviated the route of administration to IV and IT, instead of using the full term in capital letters.

Poor prescribing practice.

When the fasting error was discovered, the chemotherapy procedure was postponed from the morning to the afternoon list.

The doctor who had been due to administer the intrathecal drug had booked the afternoon off and assumed that another doctor in charge of the wards that day would take over. No formal face-to-face handover was carried out between the two doctors.

Communication failure. Poor handover of task responsibilities. Inappropriate task delegation.

The patient arrived in the anaesthetic room and the oncology Senior Registrar was called to administer the chemotherapy.

However the doctor was unable to leave his ward and assured the anaesthetist that he should go ahead as this was a straightforward procedure.

Inadequate protocols regulating the administration of high toxicity drugs.
Goal conflict between ward and theatre duties. Poor practice expecting the doctor to be in two places at the same time.

The oncology Senior Registrar was not aware that both drugs had been delivered to theatre. The anaesthetist had the expertise to administer drugs intrathecally but had never administered chemotherapy. He injected the methotrexate intravenously and the vincristine into the patient's spine. Intrathecal injection of vincristine is almost invariably fatal, and the patient died 5 days later.

Situational awareness error. Inappropriate task delegation and lack of training. Poor practice to allow chemotherapy drugs to be administered by someone with no oncology experience.
Drug administration error.

Although *An Organisation with a Memory* analyses this sorry tale in the context of system failures rather than individual fault, it is clear that many of the failings represent a mixture of the two. Indeed, many of the actions undertaken by individual members of the hospital staff could be analysed in terms of person-centred fault. But that is not the point. The systems approach suggests that we should not automatically assume that we should look for an individual to blame for an adverse outcome. What we are asking is that when an error is made, the finger should not necessarily be pointed at the doctor who made the final error. We are asking that a more considered approach be taken that looks at matters in the round, that digs a little deeper and tests the role of management and the systems that operate in the hospital. For experience shows that when one digs a little deeper, mistakes are usually a mixture of system failures and individual fault.

Although the errors committed in this maladministration of vincristine are, of course, specific to the case, they also illustrate general issues and a number of themes emerge that warrant further discussion.

Failure to follow protocols (Case 25)

The decade since the writing of *An Organisation with a Memory* has seen the introduction of numerous protocols and standard operating policies to try to improve the service offered by the NHS to its patients: protocols for the treatment of specific diseases, to stop the spread of infections such as MRSA, for the care of outliers, for the running of EDs and also checklists for use in theatres. These can only be for the good, setting in place good working practices and, therefore, improving patient care.

A doctor can take some comfort that by adhering to a protocol he[1] will be protected from criticism. In principle, a protocol issued by a respectable source can be regarded as a statement by a responsible body of medical opinion on what to do in a particular set of circumstances. But adherence may not always provide protection to a doctor. There may be some circumstance relevant to the individual patient that renders a particular protocol or part of a protocol inappropriate. A protocol should not replace good judgement.

That said, a doctor should be very careful before departing from a protocol. He should have clearly thought out the reasons for doing this and ideally have discussed it with his superiors or colleagues. He should also note the reasons for his actions within the medical records.

Inadequate communication (Cases 1, 13–15, 18, 19, 27, 29, 30, 33, 34, 36)

Several of the errors in the vincristine case can be categorized as communication errors. This is not surprising. Many errors in diagnosis and treatment can be traced back to inadequate communication either between the patient and the treating clinicians or between members of the team or teams treating the patient.

It is perhaps obvious, but it is worth stating all the same. Communication is only achieved when someone says or writes information in such a way that the other understands. It must be clear. When it is done well, it facilitates good treatment. It is key to the smooth running of all organizations and the NHS is no exception. Communication, communication, communication: this should be the mantra of all medical teams.

Although communication is omnipresent and relates to all aspects of practice, we wish to point out the following issues:

• Telephone advice – Frequently paediatricians are required to advise parents over the telephone. Such advice should be recorded in the medical notes or electronically to document the episode and for the information of other treating clinicians.

---

[1] In this book the general use of the personal pronoun (e.g. 'he', 'him', 'his') indicates, in all but specific cases, both male and female doctors, patients, etc.

- Transfer to ICU – Poor communication between departments often causes unwarranted delays in the transfer of patients to ICU with the attendant risk of a deterioration in the patient's condition (see Case 29).
- Equipment – It is surprising how often a doctor will seek some piece of equipment and discover that it is either missing or does not function. Such lack of useful equipment causes delays in treatment. Often the cause lies in the fact that staff do not report equipment faults.
- Safety net – Clear instructions should be provided to the parents of patients prior to their discharge from the ward, ED or clinic. They should be told what symptoms and signs they should look out for and be advised on when they should take their child back to their GP and when they should return to the ED.
- Abnormal results – Abnormal test results should be communicated as fast as possible, so that appropriate investigations and treatment can be instigated.
- Poor attendance – If a patient fails to attend outpatient appointments, then this can seriously affect their care. The parents of the child should be told how important it is for them to attend appointments. If a parent consistently fails to bring a child to his appointments, this may give rise to child protection concerns that should be communicated to the appropriate authorities.

Communication can be achieved through the written or the spoken word. Although it is possible to criticize individuals for failures in communication, there will generally be a systems element to such failings. Good communication is fostered by good leadership, the type of leadership that encourages teamwork and an atmosphere in which all members of a team, even the most junior, can feel confident in expressing themselves.

Poor and inadequate record-keeping (Case 3)

We have already said that communication can be through the written or spoken word. Good record-keeping should be seen simply as a subset of good communication. Full, well documented notes are a crucial part of good medical practice.

On a more general note, accurate and full records are often the only way of gauging a deterioration in the patient's condition, allowing the clinicians to change their treatment plans to treat the patient appropriately.

Lack of knowledge and not knowing one's limitations (Cases 1, 15, 20)

In the vincristine example, the anaesthetist who administered the fatal dose of the drug knew how to administer drugs intrathecally, but had no oncology experience: he had never administered chemotherapy. A doctor's care is always judged by the standard of the reasonable or responsible doctor. The responsible doctor in this anaesthetist's shoes should have sought assistance or at least double-checked what was required.

The same applies to any junior doctor who is learning the ropes. If he is asked to do something or finds himself in a situation outside his range of experience, then he must seek advice or assistance from someone with the appropriate level of experience. Again, we come back to the importance of communication within the team.

Of course, in stating that the junior doctor should seek assistance, we are presupposing that he will recognize when he is out of his depth. Common sense should tell him this, but there will be occasions when his own lack of experience will not be apparent to him. Where this happens, we should look higher up the chain of management and question whether his superiors are supervising him or delegating tasks to him in an appropriate fashion.

Poor supervision and delegation (Case 22)

Not knowing one's limitations and poor supervision and delegation may simply be flip sides of the same coin. As we have hinted, the doctor who acts outside his range of knowledge may be put in that situation by a superior who delegates an inappropriate task to him.

Poor supervision and poor delegation are classic symptoms of a system that is poorly organized and a team that is not functioning effectively. They are symptomatic of poor management at some level.

Poor prioritization (Case 20)

Any person in a busy job must learn to prioritize effectively and doctors are no exception. A doctor can only learn this skill through experience and by weighing up the risks involved in the varying decisions that he has to make.

Tiredness and stress; lack of resources

However, prioritization may not always be that easy. It is fair to say that there will inevitably be times in the career of a doctor when lack of resources, stress and tiredness will militate against best practice.

The introduction of the European Working Time Directive should help reduce stress and tiredness, but in turn it may cause resourcing problems. These are systems issues. The solutions will not be easy. If the problems become acute, then the doctor should raise them with the hospital management. But with only a finite pot of money available for the NHS, this may not necessarily bring about the desired improvement.

Psychological factors

Psychological factors play an important role in many clinical errors. We have already mentioned tiredness and stress and these and other psychological issues will be mentioned elsewhere, but only in passing. We do not intend to provide an in-depth discussion of the psychology of error. We leave that for others to do. Our emphasis is on the case studies and what they reveal about what doctors should look for when diagnosing and treating their patients (if the reader wishes to read about the psychology of error, then we would recommend Professor Charles Vincent's *Patient Safety* (2005)).

That said, we cannot escape the psychological aspects of clinical error. We give one example to illustrate the importance of this issue: another vincristine case that ended with a fatal outcome.

A locum doctor was asked to administer vincristine to a patient out of hours. He had not administered the drug previously and the mother of the patient was on hand, watching. She had watched doctors administer the treatment several times before and knew the procedure well. She saw that the doctor was making a mistake and told him that the clear fluid (the vincristine) should be put into the vein and the yellow fluid (the methotrexate) should be put into the spine. The doctor ignored her, despite her comments, and administered the vincristine intrathecally. Several days later the patient died.

Humility was what this doctor lacked. He thought that he knew best when he did not. If he had been prepared to listen to the mother, the patient would not have died.

Conflicts between system issues and personal responsibility: a healthy work environment

In our Introduction, we explained that the GMC expects each doctor to fulfill his personal responsibilities. However, he may have to do this in an environment which may conflict with these responsibilities. A doctor in such a situation will be required to perform a balancing act. If that act becomes impossible, then he must 'blow the whistle' and bring the matter to the attention of his managers. Again, we repeat our mantra: communication, communication, communication.

Despite the publication of *An Organisation with a Memory*, the NHS still maintains an unhealthy blame culture. The report pointed out the difficulty faced by individuals who draw attention to problems in their working environment. Its authors recommended that the NHS should foster a more open culture in which errors can be admitted without fear of discrimination or reprisal (though individuals still need to be held accountable for their actions).

We believe that the best work environments are those where good, professional teamwork comes naturally and people are pleased to come to work. This is an intangible element. It requires each person within the workplace to think about how he can help himself and others to work better together. If it can be achieved, then it should go some considerable way to meeting the aims of *An Organisation with a Memory* and the number of clinical errors should consequently be reduced.

Having looked at system errors, we now turn our attention to more specific areas of error, those that could perhaps be considered more person-centred. But before doing so, we wish to share some research that we have conducted on errors in paediatrics. It highlights those areas where paediatricians as individual doctors could do better. It has also helped us to establish the sort of errors that we need to focus on in the rest of Part 1, Section 2 and to determine the type of case studies that we should cover in Part 2.

Person-centred paediatric errors and their causes

We found that the NHSLA database provided the best source of information on paediatric errors. In the five years between 2005 and 2010, 195 paediatric claims were settled in favour of the claimant. The top ten most common incidents are summarized in Table 1.1:

Table 1.1 Incidents leading to successful litigation, 01/04/2005–31/03/2010

	Number	%
Medication/vaccination error	10	5.1
Delayed/failed diagnosis of septicaemia	8	4.1
Delayed/failed diagnosis of meningitis	7	3.6
Extravasation	7	3.6
Delayed/failed diagnosis of unspecified sepsis	6	3.1
Delayed diagnosis of anorectal abnormality	6	3.1
Delayed/failed cardiological diagnosis	6	3.1
Delayed diagnosis of appendicitis	6	3.1
Misdiagnosis of epilepsy	6	3.1
Delayed diagnosis of a fracture	4	2.1

The other incidents included a delay or failure in diagnosing a number of conditions including brain tumours, tumour recurrence, testicular torsion, bowel perforation, shunt blockage, Turner's syndrome and intussusception. Further events that led to successful litigation were gastrostomy-related errors, cold-light injuries and pressure sores.

The NHSLA were also able to provide a breakdown of the causes of the errors that led to litigation in these 195 cases. These are summarized in Table 1.2:

Table 1.2 Causes of incidents leading to successful litigation, 01/04/2005–31/03/2010

	Number (out of 195)	%
Delayed/failed diagnosis	91	46.7
Delayed/failed treatment	25	12.8
Inadequate nursing care	15	7.7
Medication/vaccination error	12	6.2
Infusion problems	10	5.1
Failure to recognize a complication	9	4.6
Operative problem	6	3.1
Failure to act on results	5	2.6

The NHSLA listed the outcomes that resulted in these 195 incidents. The most common outcome was death (74 out of the 195 cases), followed by unnecessary pain (35 cases), unnecessary surgery (16) and brain damage/developmental delay and scarring (both 12 cases); 5 cases resulted in amputations, 3 in visual problems and 2 in a perforated appendix.

The total cost of litigation in each of the 195 cases (including the damages and the costs) ranged from £600 to £3,044,943.

We also obtained information from NCAS which is a division of the National Patient Safety Agency. It provides advice, support and formal assessments of doctors working in the United Kingdom, the Isle of Man, Channel Islands and Gibraltar. The nonclinical reasons for referral to this service comprise predominantly behavioural and conduct issues such as poor team working and bullying. But we concentrated on those paediatric cases, where the doctor had been referred for assessment because of specific clinical concerns. Over the ten years from 2001 to 2011, there were 63 cases. The most common reasons for referral are shown in Table 1.3:

Table 1.3 Most common reasons for referral, 2001–2011

Diagnosis and management of child protection cases	19
Prescribing errors	13
Diagnostic errors other than child protection cases	12
Treatment incidents	7
Difficulties with transfer of patients to other units	6
Poor resuscitation	4
Slow response to an emergency	2

Common themes emerge from these studies (details of which appear in the references below). The most common error in the NHSLA cases was a failure to treat or diagnose an infection, particularly meningitis and septicaemia. The NHSLA and NCAS studies also showed failings in prescribing.

In contrast to the NHSLA, the NCAS study showed that the commonest reason for a complaint against a paediatrician was related to the diagnosis and management of child protection cases. This reflects the focus of NCAS referrals, which is different from that of the NHSLA; most NCAS referrals are made by NHS managers and doctors, rather than by patients.

The main causes of the errors in the NHSLA study were very much as expected, with a delay or failure in diagnosis and treatment being by far the commonest.

Most errors in clinical practice result in little or no harm. However, the NHSLA study shows that the commonest outcome in the cases analysed was death. Looking a little further down that list, the fourth most common outcome was brain damage. These observations reinforce the importance of trying to minimize errors in clinical practice. When things go wrong, they can go spectacularly and tragically wrong.

Pulling all this research together, we believe that there are certain keys areas where doctors would benefit from advice. We aim to provide such advice in the following sections. This will include advice on how to make the correct diagnosis promptly, avoiding prescribing errors, checking test results and acting on abnormal findings, avoiding errors in practical procedures, avoiding resuscitation errors and how to act in child protection cases. We shall start by looking at the patient consultation and how to identify the sick child.

The patient consultation (Cases 1, 2, 17, 24, 26, 36)

The patient consultation is, in a very practical sense, at the heart of the doctor–patient relationship. It gives an opportunity for face-to-face communication and for the doctor to build up a rapport with the patient and to win his trust. If handled correctly, at the end of the consultation, the doctor should be armed with the information that he needs to reach a diagnosis, or at least a differential diagnosis. And of all consultations, it is the first that is perhaps the most important; that first consultation will strongly influence all that follows. How should it be conducted?

A good history is essential in making a correct diagnosis. The history on its own leads to the diagnosis in over 60% of cases. Once a patient has given his account of the presenting complaint, the doctor should ask questions to clarify his understanding of the patient's symptoms. All this is perhaps obvious, but it all comes down to communication. Good communication should aid diagnosis; poor communication will hamper it. Thus a doctor must listen carefully to patients and their parents. In the words of the nineteenth-century Canadian physician Sir William Osler, 'Listen to the patient. He is telling you the diagnosis.' This requires skill and patience and can be difficult if time is short.

And to continue with the theme of listening and understanding . . . Doctors often see patients who speak poor English. Where this gets in the way of understanding, the doctor should find a translator who can speak the language of the patient. If one is not on site, most hospitals have phone access to translators 24 hours a day. A judge is unlikely to excuse a mistake caused by a failure to use a translator.

After the history comes the examination. Examining any patient may be difficult, but examining a sick child even more so. A general examination should be conducted with a particular focus on the ailing system. A doctor should try to put the child at ease; it may be a good idea to give them a toy at the beginning of the consultation, if they are very young. Starting with the hand is often a nonthreatening way of commencing the examination and talking to the child may well help to calm him down. The examination may need to be opportunistic: for example, the doctor may have to wait until the child is quiet and calm, before he can listen to the precordium. If the child is very fractious, the doctor may wish to leave the child for a while, if the situation is not urgent, and to examine the child a little later, perhaps after a feed or after analgesia has had time to take effect.

There are key areas that should not be omitted in the course of particular examinations, such as the examination of the throat in a febrile child. If the doctor were to omit this, he could be committing a significant error; he may fail to diagnose tonsillitis; he may fail to find the source of the fever. If a doctor finds a child difficult to examine, a more experienced doctor with a better, more experienced examination technique should be asked to see the patient.

If the examination is limited one should make that clear in the notes, together with the reason why.

Once the history and examination have been completed it is important to make a diagnosis or to consider the differential diagnoses in order of probability. The doctor should list the investigations required to clarify the diagnosis and to provide further details about the illness. A management plan should then be constructed. Following this pathway encourages a doctor to rigorously analyse the ailment afflicting the patient.

The history, examination, diagnosis, investigations and management plan should be clearly documented. It is also very important to note negative findings in the history and examination. The investigation results should be obtained and documented promptly. The importance of clear and thorough documentation cannot be overemphasized.

The requirement to see all patients who present to the ED within four hours can sometimes cause doctors to prioritize patients inappropriately. Thus a doctor may find himself rushing the history and examination in order to meet this deadline. Errors may occur as a result. But it is no defence for a doctor to argue this in court. This, along with ergonomic factors such as the stress, tiredness and depression, is a system issue which may adversely affect the outcome of the patient consultation. If the doctor has concerns about the systems in place at his hospital, he should discuss them with his superiors.

A delay or failure in making a diagnosis and a delay or failure of treatment are the two commonest causes of errors. The reasons behind these delays and failures are many; they include poor paediatric training, a lack of knowledge, failure to recognize when help is required and when a more senior opinion is needed, and an inadequate hospital and departmental induction to the job.

Clinicians often form a hypothesis about the likeliest diagnosis early on in the consultation. A doctor should repeatedly question this hypothesis and reassess alternatives. He should also bear in mind the diagnoses that he cannot afford to miss. So when he is presented with a febrile child, meningitis should be on his list of differential diagnoses. Meningitis may be both clinically and statistically unlikely, but it should at least be considered, if only because it is a treatable condition with potentially catastrophic sequelae.

Doctors can also make what are termed cognitive errors when they are looking for a diagnosis. A detailed analysis of cognitive errors is outside the scope of this book and the reader is referred to the references at the end of this section. However, these are some examples:

- 'Confirmation bias', where information gathering is geared towards confirming rather than refuting the diagnosis. This may cause a doctor to overlook important alternative diagnoses. In the course of his examination and assessment of the child, the doctor should not overlook symptoms and signs that may be inconsistent with the initial diagnosis and may suggest other possible conditions.
- 'Premature closure', where a doctor makes what he considers to be a definitive diagnosis early on in his treatment of the patient and then fails to reconsider the diagnosis at a later stage even if the circumstances have altered.
- 'Availability bias', where a doctor gives too much weight to his own past experience and easily recalled examples, at the expense of other and often rarer diagnoses.

Hospital protocols and national and international protocols on different conditions provide information on the symptoms that need to be asked about, the signs that need to be checked, the differential diagnoses in a given set of circumstances and the appropriate treatment plan. Likewise, different courses such as the Advanced Life Support Group's courses on Advanced Paediatric and Neonatal Life Support, and Child Protection provide very useful training in important areas of paediatrics.

As a very basic comment, it is training and experience that will lead to improved and more efficient history taking and examinations, to more accurate diagnosis and to better treatment.

Failure to identify a sick child (Case 31)

It is easy to identify a severely unwell child. The challenge is to spot the child who is not yet severely unwell, but may deteriorate rapidly, if he does not receive the right treatment. Such children will often present alongside hundreds of other children with self-limiting conditions. To make the task even harder, they may have only the subtlest of signs to indicate that they are individuals at high risk. Furthermore, it is well recognized that children's physiology allows them to maintain essential physiological parameters within the normal range for far longer into the course of an illness than their adult equivalent. The Royal College of Paediatrics and Child Health has made a DVD called *Spotting the Sick Child* and NICE have issued guidelines on *Feverish Illness in Children* to help recognize such children.

When a sick child is not identified, this is usually because early warning signs of a critical illness were missed or ignored. Therefore when an essential physiological parameter (heart rate, blood pressure, capillary refill time, respiratory rate, SaO_2 or GCS) is abnormal, this needs to be carefully explored to see if it is the first sign of an impending critical illness.

When cases involving sick children who were not correctly identified are reviewed, it is often found that the child had a single abnormal parameter (most commonly tachycardia) and that this was not acted upon. Reviewers generally conclude that the doctor did not act on this finding because:

- he attributed the abnormal parameter to some cause other than illness, for example the doctor considered that the child's tachycardia was caused by distress or that a prolonged CRT was due to environmental cold; or
- he chose to ignore a single abnormal parameter because everything else was normal; or
- he failed to recognize that the parameter was abnormal, often because he did not know the normal ranges in childhood.

To try and prevent these common mistakes, Paediatric Early Warning (PEW) scores were developed. These provide age appropriate values for normal ranges with corresponding single and cumulative triggers for review by a senior doctor.

On occasion, a child can present to the ED critically ill after attending the ED just a few days earlier. It is natural to assume that 'something was missed' at the first attendance. In many cases this is true, but it is also true that children can deteriorate suddenly and rapidly. While all such cases should be explored to see if lessons can be learned, it can equally be that sometimes, when children are seen very early in the course of a critical illness, there are no early warning signs of a severe illness.

This only serves to reinforce the need to give patients clear 'safety net' advice, when they are discharged from medical care: that is advice about when they should reattend the ED or the GP, if the child fails to get better. Such advice should be given no matter how trivial the complaint may appear to be.

Inability to perform practical procedures competently

Following the guidance below should help avoid errors whilst carrying out practical procedures.

Practical paediatric procedures require good communication skills, manual dexterity, patience, a gentle touch and supervised practice. So it is important to be aware that skills acquired during training on adult patients may not translate directly to competence in the same procedures in a child. The doctor should be aware of the limits of his competence and should not exceed them without experienced supervision (GMC, *Good Medical Practice*, sections 3 and 12).

The choice of assistant is also important – an experienced assistant is much more likely to be able to help a child remain calm, to provide distraction and to keep the appropriate body parts still and in the correct orientation, for example during a LP.

The objective should be to perform the correct procedure on the correct patient, on the correct side, competently and with appropriate consent. Pay particular attention in the case of twins and where there are common surnames.

Give adequate analgesia or anaesthesia. Be aware of the dose limits for local anaesthetics in small children. If it is necessary to tap a hollow viscus or a fluid collection, an ultrasound examination may improve the chances of success, help the doctor's understanding of the anatomy and reduce the risk of a 'dry tap'.

Prepare the trolley and instrument pack. Ensure all the necessary instruments are present. Keep sharp instruments, needles and blades inside a tray to reduce the risk of a needlestick injury. Keep a count of needles and swabs.

Ensure that the patient is adequately monitored – a small child or neonate concealed under drapes may be rendered invisible and should be monitored with an ECG, oxygen saturation meter, and an apnoea alarm, with the limits appropriately set. An assistant should take responsibility for the safety of the child whilst the doctor performs the procedure. If indicated, the doctor should check that life support equipment is present and working, and that he knows how to use it if necessary.

Good aseptic technique reduces the chance of infective complications. Empower the assistant to notice lapses and tell him to point out if gloves or instruments become contaminated. Clean the skin carefully, remembering that in infants, skin can be burned by alcoholic solutions, and that iodinated solutions can be absorbed transcutaneously.

Ensure that you understand the anatomy of the procedure. Practise using the instruments – most commonly used instruments are designed to be used by a right-handed operator and may not work optimally if used left-handed. Read the product inserts and instructions, especially if using a new type of catheter. Thin-walled catheters may become cracked if manipulated with metallic instruments. Examine distance markers carefully. The doctor should ensure that he knows what length of a tube or catheter will protrude from the patient at the end of the procedure.

When securing lines and catheters, ensure that any splints used maintain the body part in a position of function and that peripheral nerves and vessels are not compressed. Avoid encircling limbs with complete loops of tape in order to prevent a ligature effect and to reduce the risk of ischaemia.

At the end of the procedure, document the process carefully, retaining a note of the batch number and catheter type inserted. Obtain radiological confirmation of line positions if needed, record the findings and take remedial action if necessary. Remember to talk to the parents, and the child if old enough, at the end of the procedure. The doctor should explain what he has done, what should happen next, and make the parents aware of potential complications.

Failure to check test results or act on abnormal findings (Cases 1, 8, 21, 27, 35)

It is stating the obvious to say that if tests are requested, the results have to be looked at (ideally by the doctor who ordered them). They have to be considered with the care to be expected of a competent doctor.

Life at the coalface is always more complicated. Circumstances may intervene: the doctor who actually requested the test may finish his shift before the results are available, leaving another doctor to deal with them. The handover to that doctor may have been inadequate. Alternatively, he may simply be too busy to give them proper attention, with the result that an abnormality is overlooked. While those circumstances might point to weaknesses in the system, they do not absolve the responsible doctor (or his employing Trust) from a charge of negligence.

That is why it is so important that clear notes are made, pointing out the need to follow up the results of investigations.

When it comes to interpreting the results, however, the situation is different. A misinterpretation obviously might be negligent: the inexperienced doctor may not appreciate the significance of an abnormal finding, or the incompetent doctor may realize it but just not act on it. However, a competent doctor is allowed to make errors of judgement without necessarily being labelled negligent. So, in a subtle case, with confusing symptoms and signs, an expert may take the view that the notional competent doctor might well have made the same mistake as the one accused of negligence.

The subtle case, though, generally invites the objection that a second opinion should have been sought. Take the case of 'The Neonate with Abnormal Movements' (Case 21). The infant's condition was rare and the results of the lumbar puncture were difficult to interpret. But the expert has commented that a microbiologist's opinion should have been sought. He appears to think it likely that a microbiologist would have stimulated a new line of enquiry. Would the ordinary competent doctor have considered that line of enquiry?

Similarly, in the case of 'The Boy with a Limp' (Case 1) the inexperienced doctor who saw no abnormality on the X-ray is criticized by the expert for not getting a second opinion, in circumstances where there was no written report on the X-ray.

Another, not uncommon scenario is a fluctuating situation where an abnormal result comes and goes. At the time, a considered judgement may be made to 'watch and wait'. Later, with the benefit of hindsight, an expert may be able to pinpoint exactly when that policy ceased to be appropriate, with a clarity which was unavailable at the time. But that is the benefit of hindsight.

Prescribing errors (Cases 7, 15, 30)

Prescribing errors are very common. In the year 2007–08 there were 10 041 medication errors in children in England and Wales, the highest incidence being in children aged 0–4 years.

Doctors should always refer to *The British National Formulary for Children*, which is updated annually. The age and weight should always be stated on the prescription and in some cases the height and surface area are also necessary. The large weight range, from <1 kg in the case of a premature neonate to >100 kg in an obese adolescent, increases the risk of a doctor making a medication error. Doctors should be aware that the responsibility for a mistake lies with the person who has signed the prescription. The following principles should be adhered to when prescribing medication:

- Write prescriptions legibly, ideally in capitals.
- The generic names of drugs should be used whenever possible.
- Beware of drugs with similar sounding names, for example prostacyclin and prostaglandin.
- Always double-check the prescription. This is particularly important when using unfamiliar drugs, or familiar drugs in an unfamiliar setting. If calculations are involved, try to get a medical or nursing colleague to check the arithmetic. If someone questions the prescription, the prescription should be checked carefully. During working hours a pharmacist may be available to check the prescription.
- In larger children beware of calculating a dose, based on weight, that is greater than the dose one would use for an adult.
- The strength or quantity to be contained in tablets, liquids etc. should be stated (e.g. 125 mg/5 ml).
- Dose frequency, and also often specific times, should be stated and in the case of drugs to be taken 'as required' a minimum dose interval should be specified.
- Great care needs to be taken with the decimal point. The unnecessary use of decimal points should be avoided (e.g. 5 mg not 5.0 mg). The zero should be written in front of the decimal point where there is no other figure (e.g. 0.5 mg not .5 mg). To avoid confusion over the placing of decimal points amounts less than 1 milligram should be prescribed in micrograms (e.g. 500 micrograms not 0.5 mg).

- The correct units should always be used. Avoid abbreviations. In particular, do not abbreviate the terms micrograms and nanograms.
- Ensure that the correct route of administration has been prescribed. See, for example, the vincristine case above, when the chemotherapy was administered intrathecally instead of intravenously.
- Clear plans should be in place for the necessary monitoring of drugs. For example, gentamicin levels.
- Ask about allergies, and the nature of the reaction. Document the reply that the patient has given.
- Careful consideration should be given to the information that is provided to patients and their families concerning side effects. Some doctors believe that it is only necessary to tell patients of risks that have more than a 1% chance of occurring (the *Electronic Medicines Compendium* quantifies the incidence of side effects of many drugs). This is not an accurate reflection of the law (see Consent below). A doctor should always consider what would be reasonable to tell the patient and his family. For example, in many circumstances it is right to mention rare but potentially serious side effects, such as the risk of agranulocytosis when taking carbimazole.
- Doctors should ensure that the medication is not contraindicated. For example, gentamicin in renal failure.
- The doctor should ensure there are no interactions with other medicines that the patient is taking and warn the patient about possible interactions with over-the-counter medicines.
- Repeat prescriptions should be regularly reviewed to ensure that they are still necessary.
- The administration of medicines should be carefully documented to ensure that drugs are not given twice.
- Doctors should beware of vaccination errors. It is important to check that the correct vaccine is being given, that the dose is correct and that parental consent has been obtained.

Mistakes in the calculation of doses of opiates are a common serious prescription error. So, too, are errors in the prescription of anticonvulsants, cytotoxics, antibiotics and intravenous fluids. In time, computer packages and online prescribing should become available and facilitate the correct calculation of drug doses, help with drug interactions and diminish the incidence of medication errors. Safe prescribing modules are part of the undergraduate curriculum and are also incorporated into several foundation year training programmes.

Failures in resuscitation

Failure to resuscitate properly can be divided into clinical failings (e.g. failure to correctly treat airway, breathing or circulation issues) and nonclinical failings (e.g. failures in leadership or communication).

Clinical failings

If a patient's airway is inadequately resuscitated or if he experiences breathing problems, this usually indicates that the paediatrician has not involved an anaesthetist early enough. However, this is rarely an issue, as most resuscitation teams will automatically contact an anaesthetist and seek their input at an early stage.

If a patient experiences circulatory problems, then this usually means that fluid resuscitation is either inadequate or excessive.

Inadequate volume resuscitation occurs particularly in:

- severe sepsis patients, who can require very large volumes of fluid: for example 120 ml/kg–200 ml/kg of volume is not uncommon;
- burns, where the modified Parkland Formula for paediatric burns (>10% body surface area), requires 2 ml/kg/% burn in the first 8 hours after the time of injury in addition to normal maintenance fluids.

Junior doctors who have not used such large volumes of fluid in practice can become anxious and hesitant. They may be afraid to administer fluid in such large quantities. But to delay the administration of such volumes would be a mistake.

In addition, most junior doctors are familiar with the APLS principle that after 40 ml/kg of volume resuscitation, it is best practice to electively intubate and ventilate a child with positive pressure to reduce the risk of pulmonary oedema. Applying this principle, a doctor may hesitate to give more than 40 ml/kg of volume without the child being intubated or at least being reviewed by an anaesthetist prior to the additional fluids being administered. This, too, can be a mistake and could cause an unnecessary delay in providing the correct treatment. If a child is severely shocked they are most likely to arrest at induction of anaesthesia, as most anaesthetic induction agents cause hypotension.

It is less usual for a doctor to administer excessive volume resuscitation. When it does happen, it is usually in cases where children need smaller volumes of resuscitation fluid or where the doctor mistakenly treats the child's blood gas results and not the child.

Specific conditions, when smaller volumes should be administered, include:

- children with known or undiagnosed cardiac conditions (either structural defects or cardiomyopathy) who are suffering from cardiogenic shock;
- children in diabetic ketoacidosis who are particularly vulnerable to cerebral oedema following excessive fluid resuscitation;
- paediatric trauma patients, who are now managed with permissive hypotension; in such cases, overgenerous fluid resuscitation can exacerbate haemorrhage by preventing clot formation.

If he does not interpret blood gas results correctly, a doctor can mistakenly administer too much resuscitation fluid. Doctors need to be aware that the use of 0.9% saline for fluid resuscitation can itself cause a hyperchloraemic acidosis. Thus it is possible for a child's condition to improve and for him to clinically respond to fluid resuscitation with normalized physiological parameters but for the blood gas levels to show a worsening acidosis. If the doctor fails to distinguish between a lactic acidosis (from poor perfusion) and an iatrogenic hyperchloraemic acidosis, then he can administer excessive and unnecessary fluid resuscitation, and cause iatrogenic pulmonary oedema.

Nonclinical failings

This topic is a very large one and cannot be covered in any detail in this section. Suffice to say that human interactions are as important as the clinical steps in a resuscitation.

The importance of these issues in resuscitation has been increasingly recognized and is now taught in APLS/PALS courses and in simulation training. Specific examples of nonclinical failures are discussed in some of the case histories (see Case 29).

Sources of error in child protection cases (Cases 6, 33)

Failure to recognize child abuse/maltreatment

GPs, paediatricians and ED doctors must be aware that child protection cases do not come with a label. They must be constantly alert to the possibility that children brought with illnesses, minor injuries or more serious injuries may have been abused. They must remember that domestic abuse, alcohol and substance misuse and mental health problems in parents/carers are major risk factors for child abuse.

There are several roles that a doctor may have in child protection cases, some of which may overlap. He may be called on to treat a child who has suffered physically from abuse; and/or he may be asked to examine a child to determine whether there has been abuse; and he may be called on to give evidence at court.

There are two main ways in which the courts become involved in child abuse cases. The suspected abuser may be put on trial in the criminal courts, accused of rape, indecent assault or grievous bodily harm or worse. The family courts may be called on to determine whether a child should be taken from his parents, and if so, who should look after him.

Doctors, especially paediatricians, are trained to 'listen to the mother' and to believe what she says about her child. In the vast majority of cases this is, of course, the right thing to do. The difficulty is spotting the parent or carer who is lying, covering up or deliberately misleading professionals. Doctors are not trained to do this and find it hard to think in this way. It is important to be able to 'think the unthinkable' and to 'look behind what you are being told to what you are experiencing'.

Failure to act

If a doctor has a gut feeling that something is not right they should act on it. Doctors must know what to do and who to contact (e.g. the consultant paediatrician, a social worker or the police) if they have concerns about a child's safety. If they have concerns about sexual abuse they must contact the appropriate consultant paediatrician immediately so that an urgent medical examination can be arranged if indicated.

Failure to document

History

The importance of taking an accurate and detailed history cannot be overemphasized. The history may be taken from more than one person, for example each parent or a parent and the child himself, and it must be absolutely clear who the history was taken from and whether they were present when a particular incident occurred or are giving someone else's account as told to them. The details of the history should be so accurate that when the history is relayed to another professional they are able to 'see' what happened as though watching a video recording. Details should include the time and place of incidents, accidents, falls etc. as well as who was present, who was nearby (e.g. in another room) and exactly what happened. Doctors should not interview children without prior discussion with children's social care and usually the police. However if a child says things spontaneously, these statements should be noted verbatim, if possible. It may be useful for the doctor to help a child by saying, 'Can you tell me what happened?', but leading questions such as, 'Did your dad hit you?' must always be avoided.

Examination

Weight, height and head circumference should be measured and plotted on growth charts in all cases. A full general physical examination should be performed. The examination should be conducted whenever possible in a private, well lit room. In cases of possible physical abuse two doctors should conduct the examination together if possible – to confirm findings and for one to examine, measure and describe lesions whilst the other documents them. This may not be possible in emergency situations but often the examination can be repeated later by a more senior doctor in the best possible environment. Each lesion should be drawn onto a body map and also described in detail, for example 'on the left upper arm, just above the elbow on the posterior aspect of the arm, there is a blue bruise measuring 1.5 × 2 cms'. If there are only a few lesions, the descriptions can be written on the body maps, but if there are many it is better to number the lesions on the body maps and list them with their descriptions on a separate page. Each page must be signed and dated by the examining doctor(s).

Other documentation

Lord Laming in his report following the death of Victoria Climbie noted the importance of documentation of not just the history and examination, but also of the interaction between the child and the parents/carers, of things said by the child or of any unusual behaviour observed.

All discussions between professionals, for example doctors and social workers, must be documented whether these were in person or by phone. All referrals must be in writing. This may be in addition to a verbal referral which may be needed for expediency and to give more of a flavour of a case than may be possible in writing.

It exaggerates the true legal position, but it does no harm to state it: 'If it's not written down it didn't happen!' Good notes and records are key to any child protection case.

Failure to communicate

Regular communication with colleagues is of the utmost importance. Doctors dealing with a case of possible child abuse must seek senior advice at an early stage both to protect the child and themselves. When 'handing over' a possible child protection case it is vitally important to be as clear and accurate as possible. For example in the Victoria Climbie case it was said that marks on her body were not thought to be deliberately inflicted. At handover this became 'no child protection concerns' – clearly a statement with different connotations. When communicating with nonmedical professionals, for example social workers and police, doctors must ensure that they use words that can be clearly understood and that they are clear about the possible causes of the injuries. Doctors who have medical evidence to share should make every attempt to attend child protection conferences. Although written reports can be sent, it is much more likely that nonmedical participants in the conference will understand the implications of the medical findings, if the doctor is there to explain them, and if members of the conference appear to underestimate the seriousness of injuries, for example, the doctor should be able to point this out.

Summary of common errors

- Not being suspicious enough when things don't add up – 'Think the unthinkable.'
- Failure to recognize the impact of domestic violence on children in the household. These children are at high risk of deliberate harm, of getting caught up in violence and being injured inadvertently and of emotional harm from observing violence.
- Failure to put the child's needs first. The best interests of a child and his parent(s) normally go hand in hand. But when there is any suspicion of

child maltreatment the child's interests are paramount, above those of the parent/carer.

- Not referring upwards (to a consultant paediatrician) at an early stage.
- Sloppy or inadequate history. The history should be good enough 'to play the video'.
- Inadequate examination. Examination must be thorough and well documented, including clear body maps. Injuries must be described accurately. It is embarrassing to have to admit in court that a lesion shown on the left leg was actually on the right leg!
- Not admitting a child to hospital when abuse has not been excluded and it is not clear that home is a safe place.
- Not getting all previous health records (hospitals, GP, HV, school nurse).
- Not checking if the child is the subject of a CP plan.
- Failure to ensure chain of evidence. If swabs are taken from a child with a vaginal discharge where there is a possibility of sexual abuse it is essential to set up a chain of evidence. When we speak of a chain of evidence, we are referring to the integrity and history of physical evidence, from its collection to the time when it is produced at court. This is to ensure that the swab results are definitely the child's. Thus the doctor who takes the vaginal swab must place it in a sealed, labelled package, with details of the patient, the nature of the swab, the date it was collected and who collected it. When it is handed to the next person in the chain on its journey to the microbiology lab, he should record details of the time and date of the handover, the person to whom it is given and so on. If someone forgets to record this information, the quality of the evidence is affected and can be challenged by the lawyers. In some cases the evidence will be rendered inadmissible.
- Poor communication between colleagues at handovers and ward rounds.
- Poor communication between doctors, social workers and police – 'not speaking the same language'. Doctors may often think that they have fully explained the medical findings, but actually these may not have been clearly understood by nonhealth professionals.
- Inadequate documentation – especially unusual interactions between parents and a child or unusual behaviour (e.g. sexualized) in the child.
- Not documenting all discussions, including telephone calls with other agencies.
- Being drawn by social workers or the police to give a definitive opinion on the cause or age of injuries when this is not possible. All the available evidence shows that bruises cannot be dated. Some fractures can be dated but only approximately – this should only be done by a consultant radiologist.

References and further reading

BMJ Group (2011–12) BNF for Children. www.bnfc.org

Davis T (2011) Paediatric prescribing errors. *Arch Dis Child* 96: 489–91.

Del Mar C, Doust J, Glaszious P (2006) *Clinical Thinking: Evidence, Communication and Decision Making*. Oxford: Blackwell Publishing (especially Chapters 1 and 4).

Department for Children, Schools and Families (DCSF) (2006) What to Do If You Are Worried a Child is Being Abused. www.education. gov.uk/publications/standard/publicationdetail/page1/dfes-04320-2006

Elstein A, Schwarz (2002) A Clinical problem solving and diagnostic decision making: selective review of the cognitive literature. *BMJ* 324: 729–32.

GMC (2007) 0–18 Years: Guidance for all doctors. http://www.gmc-uk. org/guidance/ethical_guidance/children_guidance_index.asp

GMC (2012) *Good Medical Practice*. www.gmc-uk.org/guidance/good_ medical_practice.asp

Hampton JR, Harrison MJG, Mitchell JRA *et al.* (1975) Relative contribution of history taking, physical examination and laboratory investigation to diagnosis and management of medical outpatients. http://www. ncbi.nlm.nih.gov/pmc/articles/PMC1673456/pdf/brmedj01449-0038.pdf

Laming (2003) The Victoria Climbie Inquiry: Report of an Inquiry by Lord Laming (Jan. 2003). http://www.dh.gov.uk/en/Publicationsandstatistics/ Publications/PublicationsPolicyAndGuidance/DH_4008654

Maguire S, Mann MK, Sibert J, Kemp A (2005) Can you age bruises accurately in children? *Archives of Disease in Childhood* 90: 187–9.

Markert RJ, Haist SA, Hillson SD *et al.* (2004) Comparative value of clinical information in making a diagnosis. http://www.ncbi.nlm.nih. gov/pmc/articles/PMC1395780/

NICE (2009) NICE Clinical Guideline 89. When to Suspect Child Maltreatment. http://guidance.nice.org.uk/CG89

NPSA (2009) Review of Patient Safety for Children and Young People. http://www.nrls.npsa.nhs.uk/resources/?EntryId45=59864

Spotting the Sick Child (2011) Information on the accurate assessment of sick children from the Department of Health. www.spottingthesickchild.com

Vincent C (2010) *Patient Safety*, 2nd edn. Chichester: Wiley-Blackwell and BMJ books.

References and further reading specific to section on Person-centred paediatric errors and their causes

Advanced Life Support Group (2011) http://www.alsg.org/uk/

Carroll AE, Buddenbaum JL (2007) Malpractice claims involving pediatricians: epidemiology and etiology. *Pediatrics* 120: 10–17.

Marcovitch H (2011) When are paediatricians negligent? *Arch Dis Child* 96: 117–20.

Najaf-Zadeh A, Dubos F, Pruvost I *et al.* (2011) Epidemiology and aetiology of paediatric malpractice claims in France. *Arch Dis Child* 96: 127–30.

Raine JE (2011) An analysis of successful litigation claims in children in England. *Arch Dis Child* 96: 838–40.

Raine JE, Scarrott D (2012) Which clinical errors lead to the referral of paediatricians to the National Clinical Assessment Service? In press. Published online by *The European Journal of Paediatrics.*

Royal College of Paediatrics and Child Health (2012) http://www.rcpch.ac.uk/training-examinations-professional-development/professional-development-training/safeguarding-childr

Section 2: Medico-legal aspects

Error in a legal context

So far, we have discussed medical error in general, non-legal terms. Now we shall consider it from a strictly legal point of view. We shall look at issues surrounding consent and confidentiality, but in a legal context, as soon as one mentions error, the word negligence immediately springs to mind.

If a doctor makes a mistake in the treatment of a patient, then he or in the case of a child, his family, may decide to pursue the hospital Trust (or the doctor himself, if he provided the treatment in a private capacity) for compensation. Generally speaking, in order to win compensation, the family will have to prove that the Trust or doctor were negligent. It is important to remember that negligence as a legal concept is all about financial compensation and that the law has defined negligence in specific terms and not all errors will be considered negligent.

Negligence

Before looking in detail at what is relevant to this book, medical negligence, we need to know the basics that lie behind what is called the tort of negligence. (Tort is simply the old French word for wrong. In modern legal terms, it forms a branch of legal study.)

In principle, a person is liable in negligence if he breaches a duty owed to another in such a way as to cause damage to that person. What does this mean? In practical terms, in order to decide whether an act is negligent, a lawyer will break this formula down, looking at each of its constituent parts, phrase by phrase, word by word. For example, he will ask himself whether a duty of care exists between the injured person and the alleged defendant.

It may not always be clear whether a duty exists in a given set of circumstances, but as far as medical treatment is concerned, it is assumed that a doctor owes such a duty to his patient. The key questions in any medical negligence case are whether that duty to take care has been breached and then if it has, whether any damage has been caused as a result of that breach.

Avoiding Errors in Paediatrics, First Edition. Joseph E. Raine, Kate Williams and Jonathan Bonser.
© 2013 John Wiley & Sons, Ltd. Published 2013 by Blackwell Publishing Ltd.

Medical negligence

Has there been a breach of duty?

When the treatment of a patient comes under scrutiny in a potential negligence claim, the first question that will be asked is: was that treatment in accordance with the standards of a body of reasonable or responsible paediatricians? If it was, then the doctor or the hospital will not have breached their duty of care; but if the treatment does not accord with the standards of a reasonable body of paediatricians, then they will have breached that duty.

This test was first formulated by the House of Lords in the case of *Bolam v Friern Hospital Management Committee* in 1957. Hence the *Bolam* test.

Over the years, a body of cases has built up that indicates how this *Bolam* test should be applied. How, for instance, should we look on a case where, in a given set of circumstances, one set of paediatricians may treat a child in a certain fashion while others would adopt a different approach? Answer: it is enshrined in case law that so long as both bodies of paediatricians are reasonable/responsible, then it would not matter which of the two approaches the doctor adopted. In other words, it is possible to have more than one correct approach to treatment.

But this begs the question: who determines whether you have breached your duty of care?

If the hospital has received a letter of claim from the solicitors representing the family concerning the treatment of a child, this should indicate that the family have investigated the case and gone to medical experts who have written reports critical of the care provided. At first blush, there is a case for the Trust to answer.

In response, the lawyers for the Trust will instruct experts to look at the allegations made against it. The experts will be asked to consider both breach of duty and causation. So in the first instance, the answer to the question is that the opinions of the experts, as interpreted by the lawyers, will determine the progress of the case. If both experts, the expert for the family and the expert for the Trust believe that the care was substandard (it did not accord with the standards of a reasonable body of paediatricians), then it is likely that the Trust will concede that the treating doctors and, therefore, the Trust have breached their duty of care. But what happens, if the expert for the Trust concludes that the treating clinicians have not breached their duty of care?

At this point one may say that the difference in the two opinions, that of the family's expert and that of the Trust's expert, simply reflects two different approaches. Have we not just said that a doctor will not breach his duty of care, so long as he acts in accordance with a reasonable body of opinion? Has not the trust's expert supported the clinicians' care? Is this not enough?

The short answer is that it may be, but not necessarily. The *Bolam* test has been qualified or rather refined by the case of *Bolitho v City and Hackney Health Authority*. The judges in this 1993 case stated that although one group of so-called reasonable practitioners may adopt a certain approach to treatment, if that approach does not stand up to logical analysis, then a doctor cannot expect his treatment of the patient to be endorsed, if he adopted that apparently 'reasonable', but illogical approach to treatment. This is just one way in which the competing views of experts may be resolved. But it may come down to something less tangible: merely that one expert is more believable than another.

At the end of the day, if the case cannot be determined by other means, it will come before a judge, who will hear all the evidence, listen to the experts and decide which of them he prefers. It is, of course, he who will be the final arbiter. But before then, depending upon where in the United Kingdom the case is brought (the procedural rules differ from jurisdiction to jurisdiction), evidence will have been disclosed, meetings will be held and views will crystalize. The experts for the opposing sides will have met and their opinions may shift one way or the other. The reality is that few cases will go before a judge. They will either be settled out of court or the family will decide to drop the case.

Causation

But let us assume that the family prove that the doctor or Trust has breached their duty of care to the child. This does not automatically mean that they will be awarded any money. In order to obtain compensation, they must clear the causation hurdle. They must demonstrate that the breach of duty caused some injury or damage to their child, that it changed the outcome for the worse.

In some cases, causation is uncomplicated and straightforward. In others, it can be fiendishly complex. In the context of this book, we shall not delve too deeply into its intricacies, but hope to give you some idea of its basic concepts.

As an example of straightforward causation, take the case of a young child with a slipped upper femoral epiphysis. The doctor knows that if the operation is performed appropriately, there will be a good outcome. The doctor undertakes the procedure, but he performs it in a substandard fashion. The child is left with a bad limp. The family will easily prove causation: the poor performance of the procedure has caused the child's injury.

Causation will be far less easy to prove in a case of septicaemia. A child is admitted to the ward with a rash which the doctor should have diagnosed as being evidence of meningococcal septicaemia. Within a matter of hours, the child's condition deteriorates. The child dies. The causation question to address is: would the child's life have been saved if appropriate antibiotics and fluids had been administered, when the child presented? This question may prove difficult to resolve. Its answer will depend on a careful analysis by the experts of the medical and nursing notes to see how the child's condition deteriorated during his time in hospital and a judgement on how effective earlier treatment would have been.

Damages

The purpose of a claim in negligence is to provide the child and family with compensation for any harm done to him through substandard care. Once it is established that the Trust has breached its duty of care to the child and that that breach has caused injury, the court will move on to determine how much the child should be awarded in damages.

Clearly, it is impossible to adequately compensate someone in monetary terms for the physical disabilities they may suffer as a result of negligence, but the idea behind compensation is to put the child in the same position as he would have been, if the error had not been made.

The child will be given a sum of money which is designed to compensate him for his pain and suffering. He will also receive a sum to compensate him for any monetary expense arising from the negligence which he has incurred in the past: for example, the costs of physiotherapy.

Finally, he will be compensated for the future losses that he will incur as a result of the negligence. The sorts of loss will depend on the severity of the child's injury. In the most severe cases of brain damage, the compensation for future loss could include sums for loss of earnings, the cost of buying and adapting a suitable home, the costs of nursing care, physiotherapy, occupational therapy, speech therapy and computer technology to aid in communication. Over the lifetime of a brain-damaged child the loss that he will suffer as a result of negligence could easily be several million pounds, depending on his life expectancy.

The child may receive the damages as a one-off lump sum payment. Alternatively, he may receive periodical payments spread over his lifetime.

If, however, a child dies as a result of negligence, then the damages will be very limited. His estate will be awarded a sum for his pain and suffering and his funeral expenses. The parents will also receive a statutory sum for bereavement damages that is currently set at £11,800.

The limitation period

An adult injured through medical negligence has three years to start his claim formally in the courts. (This three-year period runs essentially from the time when the negligence occurred, but is more accurately defined by when the person harmed knew of the negligence.) Although the court can extend this limitation period in certain circumstances, if he fails to start court proceedings within these three years, he can no longer pursue his claim.

The rules concerning children are different. Children are not considered to have legal capacity until they are eighteen. Before then, a child's case will be brought on his behalf by his parents, standing in the child's legal shoes. The 'limitation clock' does not start to tick until the 18th birthday. Therefore, a child who has suffered injury has until he is 21 to bring a claim.

However, if a person lacks mental capacity beyond the age of 18, the limitation clock may never start to run. He can then bring a case at any point in his life. 'Mental capacity' in this context means the ability to run one's own financial affairs; it is different from the test for capacity in Consent cases (see below).

The most expensive cases, the ones that cost millions of pounds, are often those that concern brain-damaged infants from the most severe cases to those suffering some form of developmental delay (e.g. through an alleged delay in diagnosing and treating meningitis). It is not unusual for these cases to be litigated 20, 30 or more years after the date of the alleged negligence. This may seem strange. There are several reasons why this may be so. But the family often only discover the true difficulties of looking after a brain-damaged child when the child grows older and his lack of mobility becomes a problem and it may be only then that their thoughts turn to suing the clinical team that treated their child. Or it may be that the family's lawyer will advise them to delay the claim until the impact of the injury on the child and family can be fully assessed.

When a patient dies, whether a child or an adult, his personal representatives will have three years to start proceedings. This three years runs from the date of death or when it was known that there had been a mistake, if this is later.

Jurisdictions

The United Kingdom is divided into a number of different legal jurisdictions. In certain areas of law, England and Wales, Scotland and Northern Ireland have their own, different set of rules, as do also the Channel Islands and the Isle of Man. However, what we have said above about medical negligence applies to all jurisdictions. (The Scottish word for tort is delict, but the principles are the same.) However, these jurisdictions do have their own rules for procedure, that affect how a case is litigated.

The defence of the NHS trusts in medical negligence cases is also organized in different ways. Thus the NHSLA is responsible for cases in England, whereas Welsh Health Legal Services is responsible in Wales. In essence, however, defence of such cases is financed out of central funds, no matter where in the United Kingdom NHS hospital cases are litigated.

Issues around consent

Consent to treatment is the foundation of patient autonomy and is fundamental to the trust that should exist between the doctor/nurse and the patient. It is required for all aspects of treatment, from the administration of routine antibiotics to the most complicated and demanding of surgical procedures. (It forms an important aspect of research projects. However, consent in research is beyond the scope of this book and is not dealt with here.)

From the standpoint of the paediatrician confronted with an ill child to treat, his wish is to help that child and his parents by applying his medical knowledge to cure and alleviate suffering. That said, the general rule is that a patient, no matter what his age, a child or adult, cannot be made to accept treatment that he does not want. It is does not matter how painless, beneficial and risk-free that treatment would be; the patient is fully within his rights to refuse what he is offered. It is irrelevant that the consequences of refusal may be dire or fatal.

To put it bluntly, in legal terms, if the doctor treats without the patient's consent, he is liable in the tort of battery. In layman's terms, he commits an assault.

That is the general rule. But there are exceptions to this rule, some of which may apply to patients whatever their age and some of which apply only to children and are, therefore, of special concern to the paediatrician. These exceptions will be discussed below. But we must first describe the framework within which consent operates.

Validity of consent

A patient's consent is valid, if it is given voluntarily, and if the patient has the mental capacity to understand the nature of the treatment and has been given sufficient information about the procedure to understand its nature. In the context of errors, we are, therefore, interested in failures on the part of the paediatrician to provide sufficient information and failures to respect the autonomy of the patient, that is, ignoring his wishes. Before looking at these error types, we wish to focus on the issue of capacity to consent.

Capacity

As a paediatrician, a doctor will deal on a day-to-day basis with issues of capacity that differ markedly from those that confront clinicians in other branches of medicine. This arises out of the nature of the speciality, because the patient is a child. This feature of the paediatrician's work will have become second nature to him and need not be problematic, provided that he keeps in mind the basic rules of capacity as far as they concern children. They are:

- Children aged 16 and over are presumed to have the same capacity as an adult to consent to medical treatment (Family Law Reform Act 1969).
- Except in emergencies, the consent of a parent or, more accurately, someone with parental responsibility will be required for those children who lack the capacity to understand the nature of the treatment being offered.
- A child under the age of 16 may have capacity, provided he is capable of understanding the nature of the proposed course of treatment and is capable

of expressing that wish. Such a child is referred to as *Fraser* competent. (Such children were known as *Gillick* competent. The two terms can be used interchangeably, though strictly speaking *Fraser* competent is how such children are referred to nowadays.) There is no fixed age at which a child becomes *Fraser* competent. It depends on the maturity of each individual child. Usually, the *Fraser* test will cause few difficulties, as both parent and child will agree on the treatment and be involved in the decision-making process. The problem typically arises when a young girl turns up at the hospital asking for a termination of pregnancy, determined to keep her condition from her parents. Then the doctor will have to carefully assess the capacity of this child, to determine whether she is competent to understand.

The above points constitute the basic special rules for a child's capacity to consent. However, a doctor should not assume that just because a child is over 16, he is competent to consent; the child may lack capacity because he suffers from some mental condition. Thus the doctor should still assess whether he has capacity by applying the general rules for competency. They are in reality an extended form of the *Fraser* test. Under these, a person is competent, if he can:

- understand and retain information pertinent to the decision about his care, that is, the nature, purpose and possible consequences of the proposed investigations or treatment, as well as the consequences of not having treatment;
- use this information to consider whether or not he should consent to the intervention offered;
- communicate his wishes.

Sometimes, the very condition from which the child is suffering may affect their ability to make decisions about the treatment of their condition and deny them the capacity to make effective treatment decisions. Take the case that appeared before the court of a 16-year-old girl suffering from anorexia nervosa, who refused treatment for her condition. Although she had the capacity to consent to treatment under the Family Law Reform Act, the Court of Appeal doubted whether she had sufficient understanding to refuse treatment, because it is a feature of anorexia nervosa that patients have a distorted view of what is a normal body image and this renders them incapable of making an informed decision. In circumstances such as this, a doctor should contact the Trust's solicitors for advice and, if appropriate, make an application to the court for directions on what treatment, if any, is to be provided.

Parental responsibility

We have explained that someone with 'parental responsibility' must give consent, where the child lacks competence.

The Children Act 1989 outlines who has parental responsibility. Under the provisions of this Act, the following have parental responsibility:

- a mother – she will always have parental responsibility for her child;
- a father – but he will only have this responsibility if he was married to the mother when the child was born or has acquired legal responsibility for his child by one of the following processes:
  - (from 1 December 2003) by jointly registering the birth of the child with the mother;
  - by a parental responsibility agreement with the mother;
  - by a parental responsibility order, made by a court;
- the child's legally appointed guardian;
- a local authority designated in a care order over the child;
- a local authority or other authorized person who holds an emergency protection order for the child.

Children who are wards of court will need to have their 'important steps' approved by the court. A doctor should have a copy of the ward papers with the medical records, so that he can see what routine treatment can be offered without reference to the court.

Foster parents and grandparents do not automatically have parental responsibility. Nor do parents under the age of 16. If the parents are themselves under 16, then they can only give consent to treatment of their child, if they themselves are *Fraser* competent.

Grandparents and foster parents will only be able to give consent if authority to give consent has been devolved to them. But where there is no specific agreement between parents and someone else, that other person can give consent providing that it is in the best interests of the child. For example, if a child is injured in the playground at school and his parents cannot be contacted then it may be a teacher that brings him into the ED for treatment. That teacher can give valid consent for any treatment that is required.

For the rest of this section on Consent, when we refer to 'parents', this should be taken as meaning those with parental responsibility, where it is appropriate from the context.

Respecting patient autonomy

As a rule and just like any other patient, a child and/or his parents have the right to refuse treatment for any reason whatsoever. However, this general rule does have exceptions.

Parents refusing treatment

Parents must exercise their power to give or withhold consent for the treatment of their child in his best interests, not their own. They may withhold consent for any number of reasons. If their child suffers from a terminal condition, they may decide that he would not benefit from further painful treatment which only has a slim chance of prolonging life. Whether that decision is the right one must be judged from the standpoint of what is best for the child.

So what happens when a parents for whatever reason refuses the treatment suggested for their child against the doctor's advice? The common example is that of Jehovah's Witnesses refusing to allow a doctor to administer to their child potentially life-saving blood products. If he is confronted with this situation, through the Trust's solicitors, the doctor should apply to court for a decision on whether the blood products can be administered. In making its decision, the court will look at the best interests of the child; his welfare will be of paramount concern. Such decisions can be made surprisingly quickly. If this scenario arises on a doctor's watch, then he should contact the Trust's solicitors immediately. They should be able to make an application to the court and obtain a decision within a matter of hours.

Child refusing treatment

A competent adult can refuse any treatment for himself, no matter how vital. But this rule may not apply to the *Fraser* competent child. So in the case of a 15-year-old Jehovah's Witness, the court ordered that a life-saving transfusion be administered to him, despite both the child and his parents objecting. The order was made because it was in the best interests of the child. The lesson that we can draw from this is that although *Fraser* competence allows the child to consent to treatment, such competence does not mean that their refusal to accept treatment is final.

The issue is best determined by the court if there is time to make an application to a judge.

Emergency treatment

In an emergency, a doctor will be within his rights to treat a child who lacks capacity to consent without the authority of the parents or the court. The situation is similar to the treatment of patients who are temporarily incapacitated. Everyday, patients are brought to the ED unconscious after an accident. They are attended to immediately despite the fact that they cannot give consent. Such treatment is justified by the legal doctrine of necessity.

Information to be provided

Consent to treatment should be an expression of patient choice. But if a doctor does not give the child and their parents sufficient relevant information concerning the proposed treatment, then the choice they make will not be properly informed. This will invalidate any 'consent' or agreement to treatment and lay the doctor open to legal criticism and a potential claim. Such an error will surface, as far as the law is concerned, when the treatment for which 'consent' was given ends in a poor outcome. It is at that point that the family will complain.

In terms of the information to be given, a doctor's duty is defined by the terms of the *Bolam* test for negligence. In other words, he is to give the information regarding risks, side effects and consequences that is thought appropriate in the circumstances by a reasonable or responsible body of fellow paediatricians. Doctors commonly think that there is no need to warn of risks that have a less than 1% chance of occurring. In some cases, this may be good practical advice, but it is not an accurate reflection of the law. A doctor should always assess the parents, the child and the condition and gauge what information they require.

Child protection cases

Child protection cases often involve very young children who are not competent or able to give consent themselves. In such cases, a doctor may wish to investigate or treat the child, in circumstances where the parents will not give their consent. For example, he may want to perform a skeletal survey for new or old fractures in a child. In deciding whether he can proceed, a distinction should be drawn between treatment, on the one hand, and investigation, on the other.

If a doctor wishes to investigate the condition of the child, then he should not proceed without parental consent, especially if the investigation entails an intimate examination. If the parents do not give their consent, then he will need a court order before examining the child. But if the doctor wants to treat the child, then he would be justified in proceeding without the parent's consent, providing that he can satisfy himself that the treatment is in the child's best interests. Of course, there may be times, when treatment and investigation become one and the same thing. If this occurs, the doctor should primarily think of the child's best interests and act on this basis.

GMC booklet

As a general comment, the issue of consent is a complex area of law. The GMC has published guidance in the form of a booklet entitled *Consent: Patients and Doctors Making Decisions Together*.

Confidentiality (Case 8)

'Whatever I see or hear, professionally or privately, which ought not to be divulged, I will keep secret and tell no one': The words are those of Hippocrates. They form part of his oath and are still an important article of the doctor/patient relationship. Hippocrates simply gives voice to the fact that a full history is an essential requirement for diagnosis and treatment and the patient must feel able to tell his doctor everything relevant to his condition, even the most embarrassing and personal details, without fear that those details will be divulged to others. Updating the words of Hippocrates and putting them in legal terms, a doctor owes a duty of confidence regarding information about his patient or others acquired in his capacity as a doctor. This duty applies whether the information comes from other people or from the patient himself.

If a doctor breaches this duty of confidence then he could be sued for damages, but more likely he will be reported to the GMC. As far as it affects clinicians, the law concerning confidentiality is fashioned from a number of different sources. Primarily, there is the common law duty of confidence (constructed from court judgements). In the last few decades, this has been supplemented by a number of Acts of Parliament: namely, The Access to Health Records Act (1990), The Data Protection Act (1998) and The Human Rights Act (1998). These different elements combine to create a more or less coherent whole. What we have set out below represents a basic outline of this legal framework.

Starting with the basics, a doctor can disclose information to others if he has consent of the patient, that is, the child or, if he lacks capacity (is under 16 and is not *Fraser* competent), his parents. But consent can be implied. Most patients understand that a doctor will share information about them with other members of the health team. In other words, the doctor can assume that he has the patient's implied consent to do this.

This may seem obvious, but a doctor should, where appropriate, consider just how far this implied consent extends for any given course of treatment. It may not extend to highly personal details about the child and his family that he has learned in treating some other, previous illness. The doctor in charge of the team should consider what information it is necessary to disclose when treating the child. If he discloses information of a highly personal nature to the members of his team, then he should make it clear that the information is disclosed to them in confidence. He should also tell the family and/or the child that the information has been shared with other members of the team.

Confidentiality issues particular to paediatrics

Unlike clinicians in other specialties, paediatricians will often receive information from people other than their immediate patient, the child. Frequently, it is the parents who will provide much of the relevant history. This should not cause a problem in itself, but a doctor could find that the parents divulge information about themselves or each other that is of a highly personal nature. Though the doctor's primary duty is to the child, he also owes a duty of confidence to the parents in relation to any information that they may have divulged about themselves.

If the doctor records that information concerning the parent in the child's medical records, then what should he do when someone asks for disclosure of the child's records? It would depend on why the notes were to be disclosed. But in order to protect the confidentiality of the parent, he should ensure that the information is removed or blanked out (in legal terminology, redacted) in the copying of the notes. Alternatively, he may disclose the records in their unedited form, providing he has obtained the parent's consent.

Although the general rule is that a doctor should not disclose information without the patient's consent, there may be circumstances where he would be justified in disclosing information about a child without consent, on the basis that it would be in the child's medical interest.

For example, a doctor may be presented with a child who is seeking a termination of pregnancy but is not *Fraser* competent. Having decided that he cannot go ahead with the termination that the child seeks, because she lacks capacity, the clinician should try to persuade her that her parents should be involved in the consultation. If she cannot be persuaded, but the doctor is convinced that the disclosure of the pregnancy would be in the child's best medical interests, then he would be justified in informing an appropriate person of the consultation and what he has learnt from it: that the child is pregnant. That appropriate person may be the child's GP or her parents. But the doctor should still inform her of his decision and that he will be informing others of her condition.

Obviously, if the child is *Fraser* competent and has sufficient understanding of her condition and the treatment options and risks, then he must respect the duty of confidentiality that exists between himself and her.

Data Protection Act 1998

Generally speaking, patients seek disclosure of their records under the Data Protection Act. It is most frequently 'used' for this purpose. However, disclosure of records represents only a small part of its purpose.

To comply with the Act, each Trust should have in place a number of protocols to safeguard the confidentiality of patient information. For example, the physical paper records should be carefully stored in a secure environment. Any electronic data (e.g. radiographs) should be protected with access only allowed to those with passwords.

There are any number of 'obvious' things that a doctor can do to ensure compliance, like marking letters with confidential information 'private and confidential'; taking care over typed handover sheets, making sure that they are not left in the canteen; and not leaving computer screens on to be read by prying eyes.

Disclosure without consent

There are a number of other circumstances in which a doctor can legitimately disclose patient information to another without the consent of the child or his parents:
- Abuse or neglect: Where the doctor believes that the child may be the victim of abuse or neglect and the child is unable to give or withhold consent for

disclosure, then the child's health is of paramount importance and he may disclose his belief to an appropriate, responsible person.

- Statutory obligation: A doctor is required to notify the appropriate authorities, if he attends upon someone suffering from an infectious disease or someone who is known or suspected to be addicted to controlled drugs.
- Public interest: A doctor may disclose patient information, if he believes that the patient presents a real risk of danger or serious harm to the public. Given that the patients of a paediatrician are children, it is unlikely that a paediatrician will be confronted with such instances often, if ever. But he may come across an older child who presents as mentally unstable. If he believes this instability could manifest itself in extreme violence to others, then he may disclose this belief to the proper authorities.
- When ordered by the court to do so: A doctor should not assume that simply because a lawyer or some figure of authority, such as a police officer, asks for disclosure of the child's records, they are entitled to see the medical records. He should only disclose the records, if the child or his parents have consented or the court has ordered disclosure.

Caldicott Guardians

Each Trust and health service body should employ a Caldicott Guardian. Much of the work of the Caldicott Guardian relates to compliance with statutory obligations. His role is to ensure that patient information is dealt with in an appropriate fashion and that there are systems in place to ensure that all clinicians and the Trust generally respect the duty of confidentiality that exists between them and the patients that they serve. Therefore, he should be a first port of call, if an issue arises concerning the use of confidential information.

References and further reading

Department of Health (2000) An Organisation with a Memory: The Report of an Expert Group on Learning from Adverse Events in the NHS, Chaired by the Chief Medical Officer. http://www.dh.gov.uk/en/ Publicationsandstatistics/Publications/PublicationsPolicyAndGuidance/ Browsable/DH_4098184

GMC (2006) Good Medical Practice. www.gmc-uk.org/guidance/good_ medical_practice.asp

GMC (2008) Consent: Patients and Doctors making decisions together. http://www.gmc-uk.org/guidance/ethical_guidance/consent_guidance_ index.asp

PART 2

Clinical cases

Introduction

Having set the scene with a general discussion of error and medico-legal theory, we now come to the backbone of our book: the case studies. We have chosen 36 cases which are based on actual scenarios but which have been anonymized and altered to preserve confidentiality and to maximize the educational messages of the case. In addition to a medical and legal comment, at various points in the description of a case, we ask direct questions that are designed to engage the reader in the case and to get them to think about how they would respond if they were in that situation. The case studies are rounded off with key learning points.

The medical comment is provided in the section entitled 'Expert Opinion'. In the Legal Comment section, reference is often made to the 'instructed expert'. This instructed expert refers to the expert that the hospital or the family may instruct as part of the litigation process. His or her views may differ from that of the writer of the medical, Expert Opinion. As much as it is a science, medicine is also an art. There is often room for argument over the finer points of a case. But that does not obviate the general conclusions that we draw, or the benefits that can be gained from the reading of our case studies.

They are here to stimulate thought and encourage learning and to help diminish the incidence of errors.

Avoiding Errors in Paediatrics, First Edition. Joseph E. Raine, Kate Williams and Jonathan Bonser.
© 2013 John Wiley & Sons, Ltd. Published 2013 by Blackwell Publishing Ltd.

Case 1 A boy with a limp

Sam, an 11-year-old boy presents to the ED with a limp. He was playing football 2 days earlier but does not recall any injury. He is otherwise well with no history of recent illness. On examination Sam is noted to be obese with a weight of 74 kg. He is apyrexial. He has an obvious limp and Dr Butler, the FY2 in the ED, notes that the movements of the left hip are limited and painful. He does a FBC, CRP and ESR, which are all normal, and orders a pelvic X-ray on which he can see no abnormality. Dr Butler diagnoses a sprained muscle or a transient synovitis and prescribes ibuprofen. He also makes a referral to the paediatric clinic because of Sam's obesity.

Do you agree with the diagnosis? Would you have managed the case differently?

Sam does not attend that appointment, which is 7 weeks later and is referred back to his GP. Sam sees his GP 3 months after the initial visit to the ED because he still has a limp and the pain has got significantly worse. The GP is concerned about the length of time that the limp has lasted for and refers him to the paediatric rapid referral clinic where he is seen the next day.

In the paediatric clinic he is apyrexial and is noted to have a limp and a leg that is flexed and externally rotated. There is left hip tenderness and a significantly restricted range of movements. There are no other signs. The paediatrician, who also asks about the obesity, discovers that there is a family history of hypothyroidism and that Sam also has a small goitre and is short with a height of 130 cm which is on the second centile.

What investigations would you perform?

A FBC, CRP, ESR, TFT, TPO antibodies, glucose and an insulin like growth factor 1 (IGF-1) are done and a pelvic X-ray and a frog leg view (see Case Figure 1.1) are obtained.

The results are as follows:

FBC	Normal	Normal
ESR	12 mm/hour	<15 mm/hour
CRP	4 mg/L	<6 mg/L
FT4	8.9 pmol/L	12–22 pmol/L
TSH	62 mU/L	0.5–5.0 mU/L
TPO antibodies	1221 IU/ml	0–34 IU/ml
Glucose	5.2 mmol/L	3.5–5.5 mmol/L
IGF-1	39 nmol/L	18–90 nmol/L

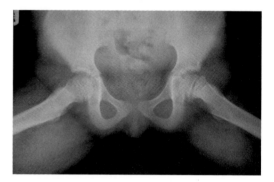

Case Figure 1.1 Frog leg view

The paediatrician asks the radiologist to report the X-rays urgently. The radiologist diagnoses a left sided slipped upper femoral epiphysis (SUFE) which is clear on the pelvic X-ray and frog leg views. The radiologist also comments that the slip could be seen on the initial pelvic X-ray 3 months earlier. However, due to an error the initial X-ray was never reported.

What would you do now?

Sam is referred to the orthopaedic team who see him later that day and operate on him the next day pinning the femoral head to the femoral neck. The paediatrician also diagnoses Hashimoto's (autoimmune) thyroiditis and commences thyroxine.

Avoiding Errors in Paediatrics, First Edition. Joseph E. Raine, Kate Williams and Jonathan Bonser.
© 2013 John Wiley & Sons, Ltd. Published 2013 by Blackwell Publishing Ltd.

Following surgery Sam continues to have hip pain, diminished hip movements and a limp and subsequently requires an arthrodesis (hip fusion).

Sam's mother complains and then sues the hospital, stating that if the diagnosis had been made at the first visit then her son would have not have suffered for so long and would not have required a second operation.

 Expert opinion

A limp is a common problem in children and requires an evaluation of the back, hip, knee, ankle and foot. The problem may be orthopaedic, rheumatological, neurological or dermatological. One should also remember that hip pain can be referred to the knee. Though it is very important to rule out an infective condition such as a septic arthritis, other conditions must also be considered especially in a child who is systemically well and apyrexial.

SUFE is the most common hip disorder in adolescence. It occurs in children aged 10–16 years with a mean age of 13 years in boys and 11.5 years in girls. It is commoner in boys (2.5:1), on the left and obesity is a risk factor.

Dr Butler, the FY2, should have told Sam's mother to return to the ED if the pain had not improved within a few days. He should also have known more about SUFE, been aware of the frequency of this disorder in this age group and of the increased likelihood of a SUFE in an obese patient. A FY2 will have little experience in interpreting pelvic X-rays and Dr Butler should have asked an orthopaedic surgeon or radiologist for a second opinion on the X-ray.

In the 10–16 years age group a frog leg (or lateral hip) view is required as some slips are not obvious on the pelvic X-ray. In confirmed cases urgent orthopaedic assessment and treatment are required as even in those with a long history of several months, an acute on chronic slip can occur which can lead to avascular necrosis of the femoral head.

25% of patients also have a contralateral slip and the other hip must therefore be carefully assessed.

A minority of patients with SUFE have an underlying endocrinopathy or metabolic disorder (hypothyroidism, hypogonadism, growth hormone abnormalities, panhypopituitarism or renal osteodystrophy) and if this is suspected then the appropriate investigations should be performed. Obese individuals, such as Sam, should also have their fasting glucose measured. A better history and examination may have led to the diagnosis of hypothyroidism at the initial visit.

Sam's mother is justified in claiming that the diagnosis of a SUFE should have been made following the initial visit to the ED.

 Legal comment

The expert comment above states that Sam's mother is justified in claiming that the diagnosis should have been made earlier. An instructed expert is likely to be critical of the actions of the FY2 in ED. Although Dr Butler examined the X-ray he failed to detect the abnormality and did not request a second opinion. The radiologist looking at the X-ray 3 months later commented that the slip was visible on the initial X-ray. Maybe a frog leg or lateral view of the hip should have been taken, as this would have revealed the problem more clearly. Dr Butler also failed to advise Sam's mother to bring him back if there was no improvement. Earlier intervention may not have cured the problem. However, an instructed expert is likely to conclude that earlier intervention would have made a difference. Thus the case will probably be settled. The claim will be worth at least £70,000 and possibly much more depending on the patient's prognosis post arthrodesis.

 Key learning points

Specific to the case

1. A limp in a child requires an assessment of the back, hip, knee, ankle and foot.
2. SUFE is the most common hip disorder in adolescence, obesity is a risk factor.
3. A frog leg (or lateral hip) view is also required as a minor slip may not be obvious on the pelvic X-ray.
4. Treatment is urgent as an acute on chronic slip can occur which may lead to avascular necrosis of the femoral head.
5. In a minority of cases of SUFE there is an underlying endocrinological or metabolic abnormality.

General points

1. A sound knowledge of common orthopaedic emergencies is essential in doctors working in the ED.
2. Even in the busy environment of an ED it is essential to obtain a good history and examination in order to reach the correct diagnosis.

3. Clear instructions should be given to parents on the natural history of their child's condition and at what point they should seek a further medical opinion.

4. A junior doctor should have a low threshold for obtaining a second opinion on a X-ray of a part of the anatomy that they are not familiar with.

5. The hospital should review its procedures for reporting X-rays.

Further reading and references

Thacker MM, Clarke MS (2009) Slipped Capital Femoral Epiphysis. http://emedicine.medscape.com/article/1248422-overview

Tidy C (2008) Slipped Upper Femoral Epiphysis. http://www.patient.co.uk/doctor/Slipped-Upper-Femoral-Epiphysis.htm

Case 2 A fitting infant

Alesha had multiple reviews by the midwife and GP because of repeated episodes of crying and irritability. She fed poorly initially but this had improved. She is the first child of her mother, Sharon, who seems to be at the end of her tether. Sharon is well, not on any medication and does not abuse drugs. The GP, Dr Robson, cannot find any abnormal signs examining the infant and he and the midwife ascribe the problem to 'an over anxious first time mum'.

At the age of 3 months whilst on the way home from visiting grandma, Alesha has a fit and an ambulance is called. She is still fitting on arrival at the hospital. The oxygen saturation is 84% but normalizes following the administration of oxygen. Breathing and circulation are stable. Buccal midazolam, iv lorazepam, rectal paraldehyde and iv phenytoin are required to stop the fit which lasts for a total of 1 hour and 5 minutes. Intravenous ceftraixone is also administered though Alesha's temperature is only 37.1°C. There is no rash, the anterior fontanelle is flat and there is no obvious neck stiffness. A FBC, CRP, U and E's, bone chemistry and LFTs are normal. A blood culture is performed and a urine dipstick is normal. A cranial CT scan is also normal. A provisional diagnosis of epilepsy is made.

What is your opinion of the emergency management?

Alesha continues to have fits overnight which require additional iv lorazepam and rectal paraldehyde. She has 6 fits in total lasting between 5 and 20 minutes. Alesha remains apyrexial but is noted to be irritable.

On the following morning on the consultant ward round it is noted that the blood glucose has never been measured. A bedside reading is immediately done and the blood glucose is found to be 1.3 mmol/L (this is confirmed by the laboratory measurement which is 1.1 mmol/L). A more detailed history reveals that the irritability and fits usually preceded a feed. Detailed en-

docrinological and metabolic blood and urine tests are done during an episode of hypoglycaemia. Alesha goes on to have pre-feed blood glucose readings which range between 1.5 and 3.6 mmol/L. Higher volume feeds are given 3 hourly, rather than 4 hourly, with nasogastric top ups and the pre-feed glucose levels rise to ≥ 2.6 mmol/L and the fits stop.

What is the likeliest diagnosis?

The insulin level is found to be inappropriately high at a time when the blood glucose was low and a diagnosis of persistent hyperinsulinaemic hypoglycaemia of infancy (PHHI) is made. An EEG shows minor abnormalities only and a MRI is normal.

Alesha is referred to a tertiary unit and a number of drugs such as diazoxide and octreotide are tried. However, these fail to abolish the hypoglycaemia and a 95% pancreatectomy is performed. Alesha remains hypoglycaemic and requires a further operation where a further 4% of her pancreas is removed.

What long-term sequelae are likely to develop following surgery?

Subsequently, Alesha has normal blood glucose levels but goes on to develop type 1 diabetes and malabsorption requiring pancreatic supplements.

At 5 years of age she is diagnosed as having moderate learning difficulties and her mother Sharon sues Dr Robson and the hospital because of the delay in the diagnosis which she feels has led to the learning difficulties.

Expert opinion

Sharon had repeated visits to her midwife and GP, Dr Robson, and regrettably her concerns were not taken sufficiently seriously. Neither Dr Robson, the midwife nor the junior medical staff took a sufficiently detailed

---

Avoiding Errors in Paediatrics, First Edition. Joseph E. Raine, Kate Williams and Jonathan Bonser.
© 2013 John Wiley & Sons, Ltd. Published 2013 by Blackwell Publishing Ltd.

history to establish the link between feeding and the excessive crying, irritability and fits.

Measuring the blood glucose in a fitting child should be standard practice. After basic resuscitation relating to the airway, breathing and circulation (ABC) the mnemonic DEFG is often used which stands for Don't Ever Forget Glucose. There is little point in performing sophisticated tests such as a CT scan, yet not doing a very basic bedside test which takes 30 seconds such as a blood glucose measurement.

PHHI is the commonest cause of hypoglycaemia in infancy. It is associated in some studies with learning difficulties and nonhypoglycaemic fits which are often attributed to brain damage from early hypoglycaemic events and seizures, and these may have led to Alesha's learning difficulties. However, other studies have shown normal development. There is also some data to suggest that infants diagnosed and treated early have a better neuro-developmental outcome. There are no comprehensive long-term studies of neuro-developmental outcomes in patients with PHHI.

 Legal comment

The Expert Opinion above criticizes the actions of the hospital. An expert is likely to conclude that the blood glucose should have been tested earlier. However, it is by no means clear that earlier intervention would have made much difference to the outcome. The lawyer will ask his instructed causation expert to comment on whether, on the balance of probabilities, earlier treatment would have:

1. saved a greater portion of Alesha's pancreas;
2. prevented the onset of diabetes;
3. prevented the neurological problems.

These causation issues will determine whether the case will be pursued by the parents. If the instructed experts conclude that treatment would have prevented these outcomes, then the case may be worth more than a million pounds, depending on Alesha's ability to look after herself in the future and her prospects on the job market. But if there is significant doubt that a better outcome would have been achieved, then the case may be dropped or settled for a modest sum.

The lawyers will also wish to look at the actions of Dr Robson and the midwife (if she belonged to a differ-

ent Trust). If their actions were inappropriate, then the midwife's Trust and the GP (through his MDO) should contribute to any settlement.

 Key learning points

Specific to the case

1. In any fitting child it is mandatory to perform a blood glucose measurement to rule out hypoglycaemia as the cause of the fit.
2. Beyond the neonatal period severe sepsis (e.g. Gram negative sepsis or malaria), drugs (e.g. alcohol), endocrinological disorders (e.g. hyperinsulinaemia, ketotic hypoglycaemia, adrenal insufficiency), liver dysfunction and inborn errors of metabolism (e.g. galactosaemia, maple syrup urine disease) are the commonest causes of hypoglycaemia.
3. PHHI is the commonest cause of hypoglycaemia in infancy.

General points

1. It is very important to take a detailed history and to listen carefully to the parent's concerns. A good history is essential in making a diagnosis and in at least 60% of cases leads to the diagnosis.

Further reading and references

Gillespie RS, Ponder S (2008) Persistent Hyperinsulinaemic Hypoglycaemia of Infancy. http://emedicine.medscape.com/article/923538-overview

Hampton JR, Harrison MJG, Mitchell JRA et al. (1975) Relative Contribution of History Taking, Physical Examination and Laboratory Investigation to Diagnosis and Management of Medical Outpatients. http://www.ncbi.nlm.nih.gov/pmc/articles/PMC1673456/pdf/brmedj01449-0038.pdf

Hoffman RP (2009) Hypoglycaemia. http://emedicine.medscape.com/article/921936-overview

Markert RJ, Haist SA, Hillson SD et al. (2004) Comparative Value of Clinical Information in Making a Diagnosis. http://www.ncbi.nlm.nih.gov/pmc/articles/PMC1395780/

Case 3 A persistent fever

Arun, a 4-year-old boy, presents to the ED with a fever, coryza and an earache. On examination he is found to have a temperature of 39.1°C, an erythematous throat and pink ear drums. A diagnosis of an upper respiratory tract infection is made by the FY2 doctor. Arun's mother is told that the infection is probably viral and is asked to return if Arun does not improve with analgesia and antipyretics. Two days later Arun represents to ED and this time is seen by a different FY2 doctor. The temperature has persisted and is 39.2°C and Arun is still complaining of ear ache and is now also lethargic and anorexic. His mother also feels that Arun cannot hear properly in his right ear. There is no rash.

Which other symptoms and signs would it be important to document?

There is no documentation regarding symptoms and signs such as a headache, irritability, photophobia or neck stiffness in this or the previous attendance. The FY2 makes the same diagnosis but this time prescribes amoxicillin and Arun is discharged.

He returns 2 days later in the evening as he has deteriorated and is now also complaining of a headache and has vomited twice. This time he is referred to the paediatric team. He still has a temperature and an ear ache. He has no photophobia. The paediatric ST1 also documents that Arun has not been immunized. On examination, his temperature is 39.7°C and there is no rash. Arun's throat is slightly erythematous but with no pus or tonsillar enlargement. His ears appear normal. He can extend his neck fully and can also flex his neck but is unable to get his chin to touch his chest. The registrar reviews Arun, elicits the same signs, and is unsure if the limited neck flexion is abnormal.

Is the neck flexion within normal limits?

A FBC, CRP, U and E's, bone chemistry, LFTs, blood culture and meningococcal PCR are performed and urine is collected for microscopy and culture. The registrar wants to do a LP but Arun's mother is reluctant for him 'to have a needle put in his back'.

What would you do now?

The registrar decides to admit Arun and to administer high dose iv ceftriaxone. The FBC has a raised WBC of 22.4×10^9/L (normal 4–11×10^9/L), the CRP is also elevated at 143 mg/L (normal<6 mg/L) and the U and E's, bone chemistry, LFTs and urine dipstick are normal. The following morning Arun has a 20-minute generalized seizure which is terminated with iv lorazepam. A cranial CT scan is done which is normal and later that afternoon a LP is performed. The CSF has a WBC count of 684×10^6/L (normal<5×10^6/L) of which 60% are polymorphs, a protein of 1.6 g/L (normal 0.2–0.4 g/L) and a glucose of 1.9 mmol/L (normal 2.8–4.4 mmol/L). Gram stain is negative but the rapid antigen screen is positive for *Haemophilus influenzae* and a diagnosis of *H. influenzae* meningitis is made.

Does this result influence your management plan?

Intravenous dexamethasone is then prescribed.

Arun subsequently has further fits and is commenced on phenytoin. He has a 7 day course of iv ceftriaxone and goes on to develop mild learning difficulties, epilepsy and right-sided hearing loss.

Arun's mother makes a complaint and later sues the hospital stating that the diagnosis and treatment where inappropriately delayed.

Expert opinion

The absence of comprehensive documentation during the first two attendances makes it difficult to determine if the diagnosis and treatment were appropriate.

Avoiding Errors in Paediatrics, First Edition. Joseph E. Raine, Kate Williams and Jonathan Bonser.
© 2013 John Wiley & Sons, Ltd. Published 2013 by Blackwell Publishing Ltd.

Meningitis is such a serious condition that it should always be in the back of one's mind when seeing a sick, febrile child and it is important in such cases to document the presence or absence of features associated with meningitis. It is not unusual for meningitis to be preceded by upper respiratory or gastrointestinal symptoms and it is possible that in the early stages of this case there was no headache, photophobia or neck stiffness. However, this should have been documented. The absence of immunizations in Arun would also have raised the risk of him having a serious bacterial infection and this fact should also have been documented at the first presentation. The FY2 doctors should have obtained a more senior ED or paediatric opinion on this child and this would be routine procedure in many EDs.

Neck stiffness can be difficult to assess in children under 1 year of age. However, over 1 year of age, and certainly at 4 years of age, the presence of neck stiffness should be clearly elicitable. When the meninges are inflamed flexing the neck in particular stretches the meninges and causes pain. A 4-year-old should be able to place his chin on his chest and his inability to do so denotes a degree of neck stiffness compatible with meningitis. Partial treatment of meningitis, as in this case, is quite common and can modify the signs and the investigation results and should lower the threshold for suspecting meningitis and performing a LP. Following the refusal of Arun's mother to allow him to have a LP the registrar should have discussed the case with the consultant. A review of Arun by the consultant may have persuaded his mother to allow the LP.

Dexamethasone has been shown to decrease the risk of neurological sequelae and deafness in children with some types of bacterial meningitis, particularly *Haemophilus influenzae*. Dexamethasone should be administered just before or concomitantly with the first dose of antibiotic. However, the role of dexamethasone in partially treated meningitis has not been evaluated. It is therefore not possible to say whether its earlier use, following an immediate LP upon admission to the ward, would have made a difference to Arun. Nevertheless, there would be a case for administering it on purely clinical grounds, given the likely diagnosis of meningitis, immediately prior to the iv ceftriaxone as it has few adverse effects. Administering dexamethasone following the LP was a reasonable course of action even though the efficacy of the delayed administration of this drug is unknown.

It is possible that the deafness may have been unavoidable even with early treatment, but the accompanying epilepsy and mild learning difficulties may have been avoided with an earlier diagnosis and treatment.

 Legal comment

An important factor in this case was Arun's mother's refusal to let him undergo a lumbar puncture: she refused to give her consent to the procedure. The Key Learning Points below state that, in such cases, a consultant should be informed. It may be argued that the clinicians could have performed the LP anyway, on the basis that the procedure was in the best interests of the child. However, this would have been very difficult in practice. It is always preferable to try to persuade parents of the need for a procedure or course of treatment, rather than to act unilaterally, and the consultant may have persuaded Arun's mother of the need for the LP. Ignoring the wishes of a parent lays clinicians open to criticism and to a potential complaint.

There are failings in the treatment provided to Arun and the lack of documentation will make it difficult for the hospital to defend the standard of care. However, the family may have difficulty in establishing that earlier treatment would have altered the outcome. The Expert Opinion comments that deafness may have been unavoidable. But if an instructed expert concludes that the epilepsy and mild learning difficulties would probably have been avoided with earlier treatment, then the case could be worth several hundred thousand pounds and perhaps even more. This would depend on Arun's ability to look after himself in the future and his prospects on the job market.

 Key learning points

Specific to the case

1. Meningitis should always be considered in a febrile, sick child as it is a serious but treatable condition.

2. Symptoms such as a headache and vomiting and signs such as neck stiffness and a rash should be sought and documented.

3. Prior treatment with antibiotics is not uncommon. It can modify the signs of meningitis due to partial treatment and should lower the threshold for suspecting this condition.

4. Dexamethasone, in addition to antibiotics, is part of the treatment of bacterial meningitis in children.

General points

1. Comprehensive documentation is very important.

2. ED departments should have clear protocols stating when a case should be discussed with a senior ED colleague and when a patient should be referred for a specialist opinion.

3. If a parent objects to an investigation that is considered necessary and that could modify treatment then the case should be discussed with the consultant. The consultant may need to see the patient themselves and occasionally child protection proceedings need to be instituted. It is advisable for paediatric departments to have a list of conditions that a junior doctor should discuss with their consultant.

Further reading and references

Meningitis Research Foundation (2011) Useful source of information on meningitis and septicaemia for health professionals and the public. http://www.meningitis.org

Muller ML (2010) Bacterial Meningitis. http://emedicine.medscape.com/article/961497-overview

NICE (2007) Feverish Illness in Children-assessment and Initial Management in Children Younger than 5 Years. http://www.nice.org.uk/cg047

Case 4 A biking injury

George, a 12-year-old boy, is BMX biking on a purpose-built track on a Saturday afternoon and falls off his bike as he is riding downhill; he lands on top of his bike. George is wearing a helmet, but no other protective clothing. By the time his friend reaches him, George is awake and orientated but complains of a painful left shoulder and stomach area. An ambulance is called and he is taken to hospital.

His observations at triage show a mild tachycardia of 110/min, but other observations are within normal parameters. He has a bruise over the left upper quadrant of his abdomen but no other visible injuries. George is given a Manchester Triage Score assessment of Urgent (i.e. that full assessment take place within 60 minutes).

What is your opinion of this initial assessment?

Thirty minutes after his arrival in ED, George's parents arrive. They find him complaining of increasing abdominal pain and looking pale. A repeat set of observations show that his tachycardia has worsened to 120/min and his blood pressure is now a little low at 95/58 mm Hg.

What course of action is appropriate at this stage?

George is moved from his cubicle to the resuscitation area and a paediatric trauma call is put out. The full trauma team attend and the call is led by the ED middle grade. George has no problems with his airway or breathing, but has signs of clinical shock. He is given 10 ml/kg of 0.9% saline. George shows no response to the first fluid bolus, but after a second bolus of 10 ml/kg his pulse and blood pressure return to normal. Trauma bloods are sent while a bedside FBC shows a Hb of 10g/dl (normal 12.1–16.6 g/dl).

A bedside FAST (Focused Assessment with Sonography for Trauma) ultrasound scan is performed by the ED middle grade and shows free fluid in the left upper quadrant but does not show any obvious splenic injury. A CT abdomen is performed while George is still in the ED, and shows a grade IV splenic injury (where grade I is least severe and grade V is most severe).

As George remains stable, the surgical registrar does not want to operate, but asks for George to be admitted to the general paediatric ward for observation. The surgical registrar confirms this plan with the on-call general surgical consultant and George is admitted.

George is transferred to the ward where he has routine 4-hourly observations. The first set of observations after his transfer to the ward is within normal limits.

Do you think this is an appropriate management plan?

Two hours after George is transferred to the ward, his parents call the nurses as they are concerned that he is looking pale again. His observations now show a pulse of 130/min and a blood pressure of 90/55 mmHg. A full paediatric arrest call is put out. George is given a further 2 boluses of 10 ml/kg of 0.9% saline, but achieves only partial haemodynamic stabilization, with a persistent tachycardia.

George is taken to theatre immediately, while the on-call general surgical consultant comes in from home. A repeat FBC shows a Hb of 8 g/dl and George requires a transfusion of O-Negative blood prior to the operation. At operation, attempts are made to preserve the spleen by splenorrhaphy, but these prove inadequate to control the bleeding and George has a splenectomy.

After discharge George's parents make a formal complaint, stating that he received inadequate care both in ED and on the ward and that this led to his spleen being removed unnecessarily.

 Expert opinion

Splenic injury is a common consequence of blunt trauma in children. The most common mechanism

---

Avoiding Errors in Paediatrics, First Edition. Joseph E. Raine, Kate Williams and Jonathan Bonser.
© 2013 John Wiley & Sons, Ltd. Published 2013 by Blackwell Publishing Ltd.

is a biking injury, followed by a motorbike injury. Abdominal wall bruising in the presence of blunt trauma is highly significant with one in nine children having a significant intra-abdominal injury. Left shoulder pain is a recognized referred pain phenomenon in splenic injury, caused by blood irritating the diaphragm. In this case, the ED staff failed to recognize the potential seriousness of this presentation as well as the early warning signs of shock. A paediatric trauma call should have been activated following triage.

Current best practice is that most splenic injuries can be successfully managed nonoperatively with even grade IV lacerations healing well without surgery. With more severe injuries there remains considerable clinical variation in practice.

However, a well-recognized indication for changing from nonoperative to operative intervention is the presence of haemodynamic instability. It is therefore imperative that patients with splenic injury who are being nonoperatively managed are closely observed. The American Pediatric Surgical Association recommends that patients with grade IV splenic injury are observed in a paediatric intensive care unit. Implicit in this recommendation is the requirement for frequent routine observations (at least hourly) as opposed to the 4-hourly observations given to George. It would have been best practice to transfer him either to a recognized trauma centre or to a paediatric surgical centre where he could have been more appropriately nonoperatively managed.

It is impossible to say whether the substandard care George received led directly to the need for splenectomy as even in specialist centres splenectomy remains necessary in some cases. However, there is clear evidence that children managed in nonpaediatric surgical centres have higher rates of splenectomy than patients managed in specialist centres.

 Legal comment

It seems that the paediatric trauma team should have been called half an hour earlier than it was. It also seems that arrangements should have been made for much closer observation of George. It is only by luck that his parents noticed a change in his condition.

So there seem to have been two likely breaches of duty of care to George. But even so, it is very doubtful whether the parents will be able to successfully sue the hospital. The reason is that, while those breaches may have caused some delay, they probably did not obviate the need for surgery. Arguments that the delay and/or failure to refer to a specialist centre had led to a more radical surgery than would otherwise have taken place would also be very difficult for the parents to prove.

George's parents have made a formal complaint. This should prompt an investigation of the systems in place for the treatment of children with a ruptured spleen. As a result, the paediatric department should be made aware of the need for frequent observations in patients such as George.

 Key learning points

Specific to the case

1. Abdominal bruising in a child is always significant until proven otherwise.
2. Left shoulder tip pain can be caused by subdiaphragmatic bleeding irritating the diaphragm and should be considered significant in a child with blunt abdominal trauma.
3. Most paediatric splenic injuries can be managed nonoperatively, but only with close observation and ideally under the care of a specialist paediatric surgical or trauma centre.
4. Haemodynamic instability is the main indication for operative management of splenic rupture.

General points

1. All trusts with EDs should have clear guidance for triage staff regarding when to put out a paediatric trauma call. This guidance should include mechanisms of injury as well as physiological parameters.
2. All trusts with EDs, who are not themselves paediatric trauma or surgical centres should have clear guidance detailing when to seek specialist advice and when to transfer a patient to a specialist centre.
3. All trusts where children are admitted overnight should have guidance on which patient groups require more frequent routine observations (i.e. HDU standard care).

Further reading and references

Alterman DM (2001) Considerations in Pediatric Trauma. www.emedicine.medscape.com/article/435031-overview

American Pediatric Surgical Association Trauma Committee (2000) Evidence-based guidelines for resource utilization in children with isolated spleen or liver injury. *J Pediatr Surg* 35: 164–9.

Bjerke HS *et al.* (2009) Splenic Rupture. www.emedicine.medscape.com/article/432823-overview

Bowman SM *et al.* (2010) Variability in pediatric splenic injury care *Arch Surg* 145(11): 1048–53.

Veger HTC *et al.* (2008) Pediatric splenic injury: non-operative management first! *Eur J Trauma Emerg Surg* 3: 267–72.

Case 5 A teenager with abdominal pain

Hayley is a 13-year-old girl referred to the surgical registrar with abdominal pain at 2.30 pm. She has a temperature of 38.1°C and vomited once yesterday and once today. Her mum states that Hayley has stopped eating solids and is not drinking much. There is no history of dysuria or frequency. Hayley has not yet started her periods. At 4 years of age she had a urinary tract infection but her mother states that she was subsequently seen in outpatients, had a normal kidney US and was discharged. Following the administration of paracetamol in the ED Hayley is seen at 4 pm and by this time she is apyrexial. However, she does have lower abdominal pain with tenderness across the whole lower abdomen.

What investigations would you do?

A blood test for a FBC, U and E's and CRP is performed. A urine dipstick shows 2+ leucocytes. The surgical registrar considers the most likely diagnosis to be a urinary tract infection and refers Hayley to the paediatricians.

The paediatric registrar sees her at 6 pm and feels that the pain is worst in the right iliac fossa. He is also concerned that the WBC count has come back raised at 22.6×10^9/L (normal 4–12×10^9/L) with 17.2×10^9/L neutrophils (normal 1.5–6.0×10^9/L) and that the CRP is raised at 305 mg/L (normal<6 mg/L).

What is the likeliest diagnosis and what would you do?

The paediatric registrar diagnoses appendicitis and asks the surgical registrar to see Hayley again. He suggests that she is given nil orally and prescribed iv fluids and iv co-amoxiclav.

The surgical registrar returns at 6.30 pm to review Hayley. On this occasion he also performs a rectal examination and elicits right-sided tenderness. He agrees that the diagnosis is probably appendicitis, prescribes co-amoxiclav and plans for Hayley to have an appendicectomy.

Hayley is seen by the anaesthetist at 9 pm. She has had morphine and this has led to an improvement in her pain. The anaesthetist feels that she may not get to theatre until 11 pm and that it may therefore be best to defer the operation to the next day.

Do you agree?

The surgical registrar discusses the case with his consultant who agrees to delay the operation.

The following day is Saturday. Hayley is reviewed by the surgical team and is found to be in pain and to have marked lower abdominal tenderness and guarding. However, due to the fact that only one theatre is operational and that there has been a build-up of urgent adult cases overnight, she is not taken to theatre until 4.30 pm. In theatre Hayley is found to have a perforated appendix with widespread pus in the peritoneal cavity. Following an appendicectomy and peritoneal lavage she has 5 days of iv co-amoxiclav and gentamicin and goes home after 7 days.

Hayley subsequently has two more admissions with fever and abdominal pain. An abdominal abscess is diagnosed by US on her second readmission and she is taken back to theatre for drainage of the abscess and requires a further course of iv antibiotics.

Hayley's parents complain about the delay in treatment, stating that if she had been diagnosed promptly she could have been operated on prior to the perforation and that this would have avoided all the subsequent complications.

Expert opinion

The triad of abdominal pain, vomiting and a low-grade temperature is very suggestive of appendicitis. Typically the pain starts peri-umbilically and then migrates to the right iliac fossa. However, many cases are atypical and, as in this case, the pain can be across the whole lower abdomen, especially if there is peritoneal involvement.

Avoiding Errors in Paediatrics, First Edition. Joseph E. Raine, Kate Williams and Jonathan Bonser.
© 2013 John Wiley & Sons, Ltd. Published 2013 by Blackwell Publishing Ltd.

At 13 years of age Hayley is old enough to complain of the symptoms of a urinary tract infection such as dysuria. One can get leucocytes in the urine dipstick if an inflamed appendix is in contact with the bladder. The normality of her previous renal US suggests that she does not have a predisposition to urinary tract infections. Following the diagnosis of appendicitis at 6.30 pm by the surgical registrar, Hayley should have gone to theatre that evening. Furthermore, the raised WBC count and the very elevated CRP suggest a serious infection and that perforation may have already occurred or is imminent. UK guidelines suggest that patients with appendicitis should not be operated on after midnight unless there is a perforation or a clinical deterioration. In this case the failure to operate on Hayley prior to midnight and the further delay the following day is unacceptable. 10–20% of children aged 10–17 years perforate their appendix and Hayley may have perforated her appendix by 6.30 pm on the day she presented. However, even if she had perforated by that time the delay in operating undoubtedly contributed to the postoperative morbidity.

 Legal comment

Hayley's parents have made a complaint. The treatment was clearly substandard and the hospital should apologize. The investigation of the case should encourage the hospital to review its systems. It should consider how it prioritizes its urgent procedures and whether it should make more theatres available over the weekend period.

If the parents are not satisfied with the outcome of the complaints process, they can ask the Health Service Ombudsman to investigate their concerns. The Ombudsman produces a detailed report of its findings and recommends improvements. This report is laid before Parliament and is accessible to the public.

If the family decide to sue the hospital, their claim should be successful. The level of compensation will depend on whether Hayley's appendix had perforated before she should have had her surgery. If the perforation could have been prevented, then she should be compensated for the pain and suffering associated with the two additional admissions and further abdominal surgery. But even if the appendix had perforated before 6.30 pm on the day Hayley presented, the Expert Opinion states that earlier treatment would still have prevented some of the postoperative morbidity. In any event, damages are unlikely to exceed £10,000 and may be significantly less.

 Key learning points

Specific to the case

1. The most important lesson in this case is that if a diagnosis of appendicitis is made, the patient should be operated on the same day in order to avoid a perforation and its attendant complications.

2. The 'typical' history of anorexia, peri-umbilical pain followed by right lower quadrant pain, fever and vomiting, is observed in fewer than 60% of patients.

3. If strong painkillers such as morphine have been administered one should wait and see what happens when they have worn off. Strong pain killers can mask important signs.

4. Although one should treat the patient and not the investigation results the very high CRP points to severe sepsis which should have led to prompt action.

General points

1. Appendicitis is a common cause of abdominal pain in children and a surgical opinion should be obtained early on.

2. The presentation in preschool children is often atypical and therefore delayed. The rate of appendiceal perforation is >80% in children under 3 years of age.

3. Predictive factors significantly associated with perforation are age under 9 years, abdominal pain lasting longer than 48 hours, temperature of more than 37.9°C and signs of peritoneal irritation. Because of the short time from obstruction of the appendix to perforation, 20–35% of patients who present with acute appendicitis have already perforated. Estimates suggest that most patients perforate within 72 hours of the onset of symptoms.

4. A number of paediatric appendicitis scores exist and some have been clinically validated and found to be a useful tool in assessing the likelihood of appendicitis in children aged 4–18 years.

5. The differential diagnosis of appendicitis includes gastrointestinal causes such as mesenteric adenitis, gynaecological causes such as ovarian torsion or in sexually active patients an ectopic pregnancy (sexually active patients may require a pregnancy test), urological causes such as a urinary tract infection and other causes of abdominal pain such as a lower lobe pneumonia.

6. It is important to remember that appendicitis is primarily a clinical diagnosis and investigations should not be allowed to lead to significant delays. In cases of diagnostic uncertainty in the UK an US is often performed. In the United States CT scans are the investigation of choice when the diagnosis is equivocal. CT scanning is superior to US but involves a significant dose of radiation. In the UK a CT scan is performed if the diagnosis is still unclear after the US.

7. The hospital should review its policy regarding the grading of the urgency of cases on the Saturday/Sunday morning emergency list. Criteria stating when a second theatre should be opened for an emergency list on the weekend, and plans on how to do so, should also be drawn up.

Further reading and references

Alloo J, Gerstle T, Shilyansky J, Ein SH (2004) Appendicitis in children less than 3 years of age: a 28-year review. *Pediatr Surg Int* 19: 777–9.

Brennan GDG (2006) Pediatric appendicitis: pathophysiology and appropriate use of diagnostic imaging. *Can J Emerg Med* 8: 425–32.

Craig S (2011) Appendicitis. http://emedicine. medscape.com/article/773895-overview

Goldman RD, Carter S, Stephens D *et al.* (2008) Prospective validation of the pediatric appendicitis score. *J Pediatr* 153: 278–82.

Samuel M (2002) Pediatric appendicitis score. *J Pediatr Surg* 37: 877–81.

Yen-Shih P, Hung-Chang L, Chun-Yan Y *et al.* (2006) Clinical criteria for diagnosing perforated appendix in pediatric patients. *Pediatric Emergency Care* 22: 475–9.

Case 6 A young girl with a vaginal discharge

Gemma, a 5-year-old girl, is brought to the ED by her mother, Sara, who says that Gemma has had a thick yellow vaginal discharge for 4 days. Despite Canestan cream from the GP it has got more profuse and her 'knickers are soaked'.

What is the differential diagnosis?

Sara tells the ED FY2 doctor that she has asked her daughter if anyone has touched her genital area and Gemma said 'no' and Sara believes her. Gemma is said to be behaving and playing normally. General physical examination is normal.

What would you do next?

On examination of the genitalia, a thick, yellow, bloody discharge is seen. The vulva appears sore but there is no swelling or signs of trauma. A bacterial swab is taken. Gemma is referred to the paediatric registrar who takes a more detailed history. Gemma lives with her mother, spends Friday nights with her father and visits her maternal grandfather every weekend but is not left alone with him. The family are known to social services but only in relation to housing. The paediatric registrar examines Gemma again and agrees with the previous findings. He then refers Gemma to the gynaecology registrar who repeats the examination, takes swabs for bacteria and Chlamydia and prescribes amoxicillin as she thinks this is likely to be an infection due to Group A beta haemolytic streptococcus. Sara is advised to bring Gemma back if the symptoms persist.

What do you think of the management so far?

The following day the swab grows gonococcus. Gemma is recalled, admitted to hospital and examined jointly by a consultant paediatrician and a forensic medical exam-

iner. The examination shows a tiny hymenal opening, which is smooth and annular (penetration impossible). A small amount of discharge is seen on Gemma's pants but none on her genitalia. A repeat swab is taken and blood is taken for HIV, Hepatitis B and TPHA, and chain of evidence procedures are followed. The swab result this time is negative. The Chlamydia swab taken in ED is also negative.

The case is referred to children's social care (CSC) and the police, a strategy meeting is held and a child protection Section 47 investigation is commenced. Gemma is allowed home with Sara, with a plan that she should have no contact with her father or grandfather. The police plan to interview the father and grandfather who are also requested to attend the sexual health clinic for testing, as is Sara.

Sara's swabs are negative for gonococcus but positive for Chlamydia. The father's swab is positive for gonococcus. The grandfather refuses to attend for a sexual health check. Unfortunately, the swab material is destroyed so that it is not possible to see if Gemma's and her dad's gonococcus were the same type.

Gemma is allowed home with Sara but contact with her father is not allowed. Sara is thought by CSC to be 'in denial' and 'trusts the child's father and does not feel the child is at risk from him'. However, some time later Sara becomes pregnant by him and subsequently has a termination. Soon after that Gemma discloses sexual abuse by her father.

Expert opinion

Vaginal discharge in young girls is a common complaint and in most cases is due to simple vulvo-vaginitis with anaerobic organisms secondary to poor hygiene. This usually presents as a chronic complaint and the discharge is usually minimal and is not blood stained. A profuse, bloody, offensive or green discharge should alert a doctor to other possibilities including sexually

---

Avoiding Errors in Paediatrics, First Edition. Joseph E. Raine, Kate Williams and Jonathan Bonser.
© 2013 John Wiley & Sons, Ltd. Published 2013 by Blackwell Publishing Ltd.

transmitted infections and a vaginal foreign body. In this case, where there were obvious concerns about possible sexual abuse, there should have been a discussion with a consultant paediatrician at an early stage. Gemma should not have been subjected to multiple examinations by inexperienced doctors. A single joint examination (consultant paediatrician and forensic medical examiner) would have been preferable. The main problem in this case was that a swab was taken by the FY2 without 'chain of evidence' and Gemma was then given antibiotics. This made it impossible to prove beyond all reasonable doubt that she had a gonococcal infection.

Chain of evidence is a legal term referring to the need to ensure the integrity and history of physical evidence, from its collection to its production in court. For example, the doctor who took the swab in this case must put it in a sealed, labelled package, with details of the patient, the nature of the swab, the date it was collected and who collected it. When it is handed to the next person in the chain on its journey to the microbiology lab, details must be recorded of the time and date of the handover, the person to whom it is given and so on, down the chain. If this chain is broken, the quality of the evidence is damaged and is open to challenge. In some cases the evidence will be rendered inadmissible.

It is unfortunate that Gemma's swab material was destroyed as it was processed as a routine sample. Had it been saved it might have been possible to show that Gemma's and her father's gonococcus were of the same type and the case could then have been resolved much more quickly.

 ## Legal comment

It is difficult to secure a conviction for child abuse without very reliable evidence. The standard of proof in the criminal courts is 'beyond reasonable doubt', so that a jury has to be 'sure' of the defendant's guilt. Without the swab material, the only evidence is the testimony of Gemma herself. If she is interviewed it will be by trained police officers. A recording of that interview could be used as evidence at trial. The Crown Prosecution Service will have to weigh up the strength of the evidence overall before deciding whether to prosecute. In this case, the decision is likely to be that the evidence is simply not strong enough.

The standard of proof for civil proceedings is lower and it certainly appears, on the balance of probabilities, that Gemma has been abused by her father and her mother Sara has failed to protect her. However, this is a matter for the family judge to decide. Gemma is now likely to be placed in short-term foster care, with regular contact with her parents, while enquiries are made in the course of child care proceedings about what future arrangements are in Gemma's best interests. If Sara acknowledges that she has failed and accepts that the father is not to be trusted, then there is a chance that Gemma will be restored to Sara. Otherwise, Gemma is likely to be placed in long-term foster care (the prospects for adoption of a child this age and with this history are not as good as for a younger child).

As for the doctors in the hospital, they have clearly not managed the case at all well. Gemma was examined three times before she was seen by a consultant, and then important evidence was compromised. The doctors appear not to be familiar with child protection guidelines. Therefore an investigation needs to be conducted into how this has happened, and steps need to be taken to improve awareness of and adherence to local procedures.

 ## Key learning points

Specific to the case
1. Possible sexual abuse cases should be discussed with a consultant paediatrician at an early stage.
2. Multiple assessments/examinations by a series of junior doctors are intrusive and not helpful.
3. A bloody vaginal discharge should always be taken seriously and may be due to trauma (accidental or nonaccidental), a foreign body, sexually transmitted infection, pubertal abnormalities or a tumour.
4. In a case of suspected child sexual abuse, chain of evidence procedures for swabs need to be followed.

General points
1. 'Vaginal discharge' in young girls is often not vaginal but due to low-grade vulval infection with anaerobes. This does not require antibiotic treatment.
2. Girls between the age of one year and puberty are unlikely to have a fungal/thrush infection of the vagina/vulva as the vaginal pH is not appropriate.
3. Persistent, profuse, offensive, green or bloody discharge needs full assessment and investigation. Gonorrhoea in children is almost always due to sexual abuse. The incubation period is 3–7 days.

Transmission requires intimate contact with epithelial or mucous secreting cells. The organism dies within one hour of being out of the body.

4. All doctors should familiarize themselves with local child protection guidelines which should cover what to do in cases of possible sexual abuse and how to organize chain of evidence samples.

Further reading and references

NICE (2009) Clinical Guideline 89: When to Suspect Child Maltreatment.

DCSF (2006) What to Do if You Are Worried a Child is Being Abused.

Hobbs CJ, Wynne JM, Hanks HG (1993) *Child Abuse and Neglect: A Clinician's Handbook.* Edinburgh: Churchill Livingstone.

Royal College of Pathologists Working Group and Adolescent Special Interest Group of the Medical Society for the Study of Venereal Diseases (2005) National Guidelines on a Standardized Proforma for 'Chain of Evidence' Specimen Collection and on Retention and Storage of Specimens Relating to the Management of Suspected Sexually Transmitted Infections in Children and Young People for Medicolegal Purposes.

Case 7 An iatrogenic problem

Andreas, a 6-day-old preterm infant born at 33 weeks gestation, is recovering from the respiratory distress syndrome and Group B streptococcal (GBS) sepsis. However, he remains on oxygen and has renal failure which developed as a complication of his septicaemia but which is improving. His potassium is raised at 6.7 mmol/L (3.5–5.5 mmol/L), his urea is 17.2 mmol/L (1.0–5.0 mmol/L) and his creatinine is 202 μmol/L (24–112 μmol/L). He is normotensive. The night shift registrar discusses the treatment of the hyperkalaemia with the consultant on call who suggests intravenous salbutamol. The registrar prescribes 4 mg/kg iv over 5 minutes and repeats the potassium 3 hours later, at which time it has fallen to 6.3 mmol/L.

What do you think of the treatment so far?

The following morning, a Saturday, the day shift registrar, Dr McKenzie, who is close to completing her registrar training, is told by the nursing staff that Andreas has deteriorated. She examines him and notes that he is tachycardic at 212 beats/minute, hypertensive at 82/54 mmHg and appears to be stiff. Dr McKenzie reviews Andreas' medications and notes that he was given 4 mg/kg of salbutamol instead of 4 mcg/kg, 1000 times the appropriate dose.

What would you do now?

Dr McKenzie immediately contacts the National Poisons Centre who inform her that tachycardia, hypertension and muscle stiffness can be caused by a salbutamol overdose. They state that the half life is 4–6 hours but may be slightly longer in a preterm infant in renal failure (salbutamol is partly renally excreted). They suggest that Andreas remains in intensive care, with close monitoring for arrhythmias and of his serum potassium level. As 8 hours have elapsed since the dose was given, which is likely to equate to more than 1 half life, they suggest conservative, symptomatic management and that Andreas should improve over the next 24–48 hours.

Dr McKenzie contacts Andreas' parents and asks them to come to the hospital, explaining that the infant has had too high a dose of a medication given to decrease the raised potassium level. She sees both parents on her own. They are extremely angry, shout abuse at her and threaten to call their lawyer and sue the hospital during a heated discussion. Dr McKenzie then calls the consultant who comes in and also discusses the overdose with the parents together with the neonatal sister. The consultant also contacts the consultant neonatologist at the regional neonatal unit who echoes the advice of the Poisons Centre. The consultant also informs the manager on call and arranges to discuss the case with the doctor who prescribed the salbutamol and the nurse who actually gave the injection. He also reports this adverse event using the hospital's online incident reporting system.

Andreas remains unwell for 48 hours, during which time he is closely monitored. Fortunately, the tachycardia settles, there are no other arrhythmias, he does not develop hypokalaemia, and he gradually improves.

Following discharge from hospital Andreas remains well.

One year later, the parents complain to the hospital and subsequently sue due to the severe distress that Andreas suffered because of the overdose, including the multiple painful additional blood tests.

Expert opinion

Hyperkalaemia requiring treatment is rare in general paediatrics and neonatology. When using unfamiliar drugs, or familiar drugs in an unfamiliar setting, the dose should be double checked by the doctor and ideally also double checked with another doctor or a senior nurse. Salbutamol is very frequently used in childhood asthma when the dose, when using nebulizers, is in milligrams and it is this that led to the error. Fortunately for the doctor, salbutamol is a very safe drug.

Avoiding Errors in Paediatrics, First Edition. Joseph E. Raine, Kate Williams and Jonathan Bonser.
© 2013 John Wiley & Sons, Ltd. Published 2013 by Blackwell Publishing Ltd.

Though Dr McKenzie, the registrar who discovered this error, was close to the completion of her paediatric training, she should have told the consultant about the error as soon as she had finished discussing the case with the Poisons Centre. Consultants are more experienced at talking to parents about errors and will also know more about the procedures that need to be followed. In cases such as this the parents should be seen by a consultant together with a senior nurse; the manager on call should be contacted and may wish to inform the hospital's chief executive. The doctor who prescribed the salbutamol should be contacted to discuss the error and in some cases may need counselling. The nurse who gave the injection should also be spoken to. In the case of parents who threaten to contact the media, the hospital's Public Relations officer may need to be informed. The hospital's legal advisor may also need to be contacted.

Although difficult to quantify, Andreas probably suffered moderate rather than severe discomfort during the 2 days that he was unwell and more closely monitored.

 Legal comment

This case is clearly indefensible. However, Andreas was not seriously affected by the mistake. The case should be settled as quickly as possible. A year has passed since the incident. It may be appropriate to call a meeting with the family to discuss the case. This would be an opportunity to show what lessons have been learned, and to offer an apology and compensation.

The value of the claim will be low, in the region of £1000–£2000.

Further reading and references

Medical Protection Society (2010) Medication Errors in Common Problems: Managing the Risks in Hospital Practice. http://www.medicalprotection.org/uk/booklets/common-problems-hospital/medication-errors

NPSA (2009) Review of Patient Safety for Children and Young People. http://www.nrls.npsa.nhs.uk/resources/?EntryId45=59864

 Key learning points

Specific to the case

1. All drug doses should be double checked. This is particularly important when unfamiliar drugs are used. In this case, a familiar drug was used in an unfamiliar setting and this also requires careful double checking. It is wise in such cases to check the dose with a colleague. Doses, which are frequently per kilogram, can vary enormously in children. It is very important to check that that the correct units have been used and that the decimal point is in the correct place. The word micrograms should always be written in full to avoid confusion with mg (milligrams). During normal working hours pharmacists should also be available to support and check doctors' prescribing.

2. When a serious error has occurred the consultant should be informed as soon as possible. It is best if the consultant talks to the parents, whenever possible, with a senior nurse also in attendance. The consultant is also more likely to be familiar with the necessary procedures that need to be followed after an error has happened.

General points

1. Hospitals should review their procedures for checking drug dosages, especially out of hours when there is less staff and when pharmacists are not available. In time, computer packages will become available that will facilitate the correct calculation of drug dosages.

2. Hospitals should ensure that they have clear guidelines on the procedures that need following when an error has occurred.

Case 8 An infant with a large head

Jose, a 17-month-old boy, is referred by the GP to the paediatric clinic where he is seen by the registrar. Jose's parents have been concerned for 2 months that there may be something wrong with his eyes. They are also worried because he is not walking yet, though he is pulling to stand. His head is noted to be big, on the 98th centile. The anterior fontanelle is almost closed. His weight is on the 25th centile. Jose's length cannot be measured as he will not lie still. Examination is difficult as he is uncooperative. The registrar is unsure if there is a squint as Jose will not keep his head still. The rest of the examination is normal and Jose seems generally well.

What would you do?

The registrar feels that Jose will walk imminently. He arranges a follow-up appointment for 3 months time and reassures Jose's parents that things should improve.

Jose is reviewed at 20 months of age. He is still not walking and can only say three words. He seems to have difficulty looking upwards. Jose's head circumference is now well above the 99th centile. Inspection of the parent-held record reveals that Jose's head circumference tracked along the 50th centile from birth until 14 months of age.

What would you do now?

The registrar is concerned about the enlarging head circumference, the developmental delay and the eye signs and arranges a MRI scan for the following week. Jose's parents are advised that their son will need sedation to remain still for the scan.

They attend the day unit on the morning of the scan. Unfortunately, due to a misunderstanding about the length of fasting for sedation and because Jose cannot be successfully sedated, he misses his time slot. The scan is therefore rescheduled for 3 weeks time, on which occasion it is successfully performed.

Two weeks after the scan, a copy of the report reaches the in-tray of the consultant paediatrician. The MRI shows obstructive hydrocephalus, with enlargement of the lateral and third ventricles, which appears to be due to a mass in the pineal gland.

The family are called in to the hospital to be informed of the result. Jose's mother attends alone. The consultant explains that Jose may have a brain tumour and needs an urgent referral to a neurosurgical centre for further assessment. The mother states that after 5 years of marriage she is now separated from her husband and that she does not want her husband to be told about their son's condition.

How would you respond to the mother's wishes?

The consultant successfully persuades Jose's mother that the information should be shared with his father.

Jose undergoes neurosurgery where a third ventriculostomy is performed and a biopsy is taken. Histology reveals that this is a benign pineal tumour. Two further operations are required to remove residual tumour. Jose remains under follow-up by the neurosurgeons and is also seen by the community paediatricians because of his developmental delay. He has significant visual impairment, which may be permanent, due to direct tumour compression of the midbrain.

Jose's parents complain, stating that had the diagnosis been made earlier then Jose would have required fewer operations and would have developed better with less visual impairment.

Expert opinion

The signs of a brain tumour can be particularly difficult to detect in infants. A persistent visual abnormality (lasting more than 2 weeks) should be further investigated. A young and uncooperative child can be difficult to assess. In this case Jose's parents had been

Avoiding Errors in Paediatrics, First Edition. Joseph E. Raine, Kate Williams and Jonathan Bonser.
© 2013 John Wiley & Sons, Ltd. Published 2013 by Blackwell Publishing Ltd.

concerned about a visual abnormality for 2 months. The registrar should have sought the opinion of his consultant or should have obtained an opinion from an ophthalmologist.

Single isolated growth measurements can be difficult to interpret. Measurements should be compared with previous records. If the registrar had checked the parent-held child health record for these he would have realized earlier that the head circumference had increased markedly (and was out of proportion to the weight) and this would have prompted further investigation at an earlier stage, looking for a brain tumour or hydro-cephalus. At 18 months of age, a child should be walking. Many children who don't walk at 18 months will walk within a couple of months and be normal. However, not walking at 18 months merits investigation and the registrar should have considered reviewing Jose sooner.

Clear communication is extremely important but unfortunately poor communication led to Jose not being fasted properly and to a 3 week delay in the scan. Whenever an investigation is ordered, it should be ensured that the result is followed up in a timely manner. This very abnormal result should have been communicated on the day of reporting by the radiologist to the paedi-atric team. The reporting and communication of results within the hospital was suboptimal and led to further delays.

Pineal tumours are rare in children but commonly present with visual disturbances. The classical finding in pineal tumours is Perinaud's syndrome where there is loss of upward gaze in combination with pupils that are dilated and nonreactive to light.

Legal comment

A succession of mistakes by the hospital staff may have led to a delay of more than 4 months in Jose being seen by a neurosurgeon.

When Jose first presented, would an ordinary, competent paediatric registrar have sought a second opinion? If so, what would that second opinion have probably recommended? If there was a mistake at this point, it has led to a 3-month delay.

Even if (which is doubtful) an argument can be made in defence of the registrar's decision to follow up in 3 months, Jose's parents will probably allege that the hospital failed to inform the mother of the need for fasting before the MRI scan. This led to a further 3-week delay. Maybe most of the damage occurred during these 3 weeks.

The hospital will then have to investigate who told what to Jose's mother. Was the advice given in writing?

Or is it a case of one person's word against another? If it can be shown that in fact the mother was given clear advice, then the hospital could argue that it was the mother's own negligence that led to this (perhaps crucial) delay.

But, it would be argued, why did it take 3 weeks in this urgent case to get another MRI slot? Should the case not have been given a higher priority?

The following 2 weeks delay, while the radiologist's report got to the consultant paediatrician, appears particularly indefensible. Maybe it was during this period that the tumour inflicted most of the damage.

The hospital may have difficulty in defending this case, unless they can show that the damage was done before Jose first presented and, therefore, that earlier treatment would not have altered the outcome. An expert in causation would cast light on this question.

 Key learning points

Specific to the case

1. Young infants, who have open fontanelles, may not show symptoms of raised intracranial pressure as the head is still able to expand. Measurement of the head circumference and *comparison with previous readings* is therefore important in children under 2 years of age.

2. A proper visual examination includes assessment of pupillary responses, acuity, visual fields, eye movements and optic disc appearances. Abnormalities in any of these can be present with a brain tumour. Up to 70% of children have a visual problem when diagnosed with a brain tumour. If there are concerns about a visual abnormality and a paediatrician is unable to perform a full visual assessment, a referral to an ophthalmologist should be made.

3. Squints are common in babies up to 2 months of age due to delayed visual maturation. After this age, a new onset nonparalytic squint should be referred for an ophthalmological opinion for an early assessment to prevent problems with loss of binocular vision, amblyopia and the need for surgery. A paralytic squint is an indication for an urgent brain scan.

4. Guidelines are available to aid the diagnosis of brain tumours in children. They include recommendations on the appropriate timescales for referral and imaging. They recommend that if a scan is cancelled due to failed sedation, arrangements are made for a repeat scan within a week. The findings should be discussed with the family within 1 week.

5. A national campaign entitled 'Headsmart – be brain tumour aware' was launched in June 2011, aiming to increase awareness of childhood brain tumours amongst clinicians and the public.

General points

1. Hospitals should have measures in place to ensure that investigation results are promptly communicated to the relevant clinician.

2. As the parents were married when Jose was born, they both have parental responsibility and therefore should both be aware of his condition.

Further reading and references

HeadSmart (2011) HeadSmart – Be Brain Tumour Aware Campaign. http://www.headsmart.org.uk

Royal College of Paediatrics and Child Health (2010) The Diagnosis of Brain Tumours in Children. http://www.rcpch.ac.uk/sites/default/files/Diagnosis%20of%20Brain%20Tumours%20in%20Children%20Guideline%20-%20Full%20report.pdf

Case 9 An infant with bloody diarrhoea

Jamie, an 8-month-old infant, is referred to the paediatric rapid referral clinic with a 24-hour history of vomiting and diarrhoea. Diane, his mother, reports that there is blood in the stool. There is no history of travel or of contact with anyone with diarrhoea. On examination Jamie has a temperature of 37.8°C and appears lethargic. He is not dehydrated and there are no abdominal signs.

What is your differential diagnosis and what investigations would you do?

The registrar considers the differential diagnosis to be gastroenteritis, intussusception or haemolytic uraemic syndrome (HUS). He orders a FBC, U and E's and a blood culture, stool for virology and bacteriology, urine for microscopy and culture and arranges for Jamie to be admitted.

On the ward Jamie is noted to be lethargic with intermittent bouts of whimpering. He has a poor appetite and has a bilious vomit. The FBC and U and E's are normal and the urine dipstick is clear, ruling out a diagnosis of HUS. An iv infusion is commenced with maintenance fluids.

Overnight, Diane's concerns prompt a review by the registrar. Jamie still has a low grade fever and is very lethargic and the registrar orders a complete septic screen including a LP but excluding a CXR. The FBC shows a WBC count that is slightly raised at 17×10^9/L (normal 4–11 $\times 10^9$/L), but the U and E's, LP and urine dipstick are normal. Intravenous ceftriaxone is commenced. The following morning, a Saturday, Jamie is reviewed by the consultant. He has had two further bilious vomits overnight but there has been no diarrhoea or blood in the stool since admission and there are no abdominal signs. The consultant considers doing an abdominal US but as the consultant radiologist on call is not one of those with a paediatric interest and as Jamie has not got an abdominal mass, the consultant does not pursue this option. Diane is told that Jamie has gastroenteritis.

Do you agree with the consultant's view?

Later that afternoon Diane requests a further review as she feels her child is getting worse. The registrar sees Jamie and thinks that there may be a mass on the right side of the abdomen and orders an US. The consultant radiologist states that he has little experience with abdominal US in children but is willing to do the US. The US demonstrates an intussusception (Case Figure 9.1).

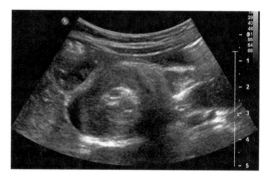

Case Figure 9.1 A transverse US of an intussusception demonstrating the target appearance of the intussusception. The outer dark ring represents the outer bowel wall surrounding the inner loop of bowel which is intussuscepting into it.

What would you do now?

Jamie has a nasogastric tube inserted and has his stomach emptied. The antibiotic regimen is changed to iv penicillin, gentamicin and metronidazole and he proceeds to have a successful hydrostatic reduction that evening in a paediatric surgery unit. However, the symptoms recur the next day and a further hydrostatic reduction is required. Jamie is discharged the following day and remains well on follow-up.

Diane requests the notes and then makes a complaint. She states that as an intussusception was mentioned in the initial differential diagnosis an US should have been done immediately, that the diagnosis took too long and that Jamie had an unnecessary LP.

Avoiding Errors in Paediatrics, First Edition. Joseph E. Raine, Kate Williams and Jonathan Bonser.
© 2013 John Wiley & Sons, Ltd. Published 2013 by Blackwell Publishing Ltd.

Expert opinion

The initial differential diagnosis is correct and gastroenteritis is much commoner than intussusception. Intussusception usually occurs in children aged 3 months to 3 years, with most being 5–10 months of age, and is the commonest cause of intestinal obstruction in this age group. The typical triad which consists of vomiting, colicky abdominal pain and loose stool with blood only occurs in a third of patients, so cases are frequently atypical. Some patients have blood and mucous mixed in the stool leading to the description of redcurrant jelly stool. Though in most patients intermittent abdominal pain is followed by lethargy, some patients present with lethargy, as in this case. Jamie's 'whimpering' is likely to have been due to pain. Initially the vomiting is nonbilious but as the disease progresses and intestinal obstruction occurs the vomiting becomes bilious. The presence of bilious vomiting, in any child, should be assumed to be due to a surgical cause until proven otherwise and should have prompted the registrar to consider bowel obstruction secondary to an intussusception and to order an US on the day of admission. In some patients a vertical, sausage shaped mass, usually in the upper right quadrant of the abdomen as most intussusceptions are ileo-colic, can be felt. However, this mass may be difficult to palpate and can be a late sign.

The twice-daily reviews are commendable, but it is regrettable that they did not lead to the correct diagnosis. The low-grade fever and lethargy understandably prompted a septic screen due to concerns such as gastroenteritis with a secondary septicaemia, but the registrar should have considered the more likely diagnosis of an intussusception.

An AXR may have been performed by some doctors. It can show a paucity of gas on the right side of the abdomen, the intussusception mass, an obstructive pattern or a perforation. However, it may also be normal, especially in the early stages, and the investigation of choice is an US.

Because an intussusception can lead to bowel obstruction, infarction, peritonitis and septicaemia investigation is urgent and the fact that the radiologist on call was not one with special expertise in paediatrics should not have been allowed to delay the investigation of this child. The consultant paediatrician should have discussed Jamie's case with the consultant radiologist on call. Had the radiologist stated that he was not able to perform a paediatric US then arrangements should have been made to transfer Jamie to a paediatric surgery

unit. It is fortunate that Jamie avoided surgery. Earlier diagnosis may have alleviated the need for a second hydrostatic reduction, diminished Jamie's morbidity and prevented unnecessary investigations such as the LP.

 Legal comment

There was a short delay in appropriately treating Jamie. This does not seem to have had any major effect on his recovery. However, his mother's complaint is justified. An US should have been performed earlier. As explained in the Key Learning Points below, guidelines should be put in place to determine what should happen in cases such as this, where a specialist paediatric radiologist is not available. If the mother pursues a claim for compensation, the damages would be minimal, probably no more than a few hundred pounds.

 Key learning points

Specific to the case

1. Intussusception should be considered in any child aged 3 months to 3 years with bloody stool.
2. An intussusception can present atypically eg with lethargy.
3. Bilious vomiting in a child should be assumed to be due to a surgical cause until proven otherwise.
4. The best-known sign, the sausage-shaped abdominal mass, may be a late sign.
5. Due to the seriousness and urgency of the situation there should be a low threshold for carrying out an US, which is the key investigation.

General points

1. The absence of the most appropriate medical personnel, in this case a consultant radiologist with paediatric experience, should not lead to a delay in the ordering of urgent investigations. In such cases alternative arrangements, such as a transfer to a paediatric surgery centre, should be made and there should be clear guidelines regarding paths of referral.

Further reading and reference

Blanco FC, Chahine AA (2010) Intussusception. http://emedicine.medscape.com/article/930708-overview

Case 10 An infant with persistent jaundice

Estelle, a female infant, born at 34 weeks gestation, weighing 1.75 kg is the first of dichorionic, diamniotic twin girls. It is the mother's first pregnancy. Estelle's mother is of African ethnicity, and her father is Caucasian. Estelle is born by Caesarean section and is in good condition at birth. She receives intramuscular vitamin K. She is initially nasogastrically fed with expressed breast milk.

At 4 days of age, Estelle is noted to be jaundiced, with a serum total bilirubin of 270 μmol/L, and requires phototherapy for 2 days. Her blood group is A, Rhesus D positive, DAT negative.

She is discharged home aged 10 days, still partially nasogastrically fed, weighing 2.2 kg (on the 25th centile for gestation). She is minimally jaundiced.

At 3 weeks of age, Estelle presents to her GP with vomiting after feeds. Her weight is static at 2.2 kg and she is slightly jaundiced.

What other information do you need?
What is your differential diagnosis?

The GP diagnoses gastro-oesophageal reflux, and prescribes infant Gaviscon with feeds. The GP notes the jaundice, but as it is less than previously and mild she is not concerned.

What follow-up is required?

At 12 weeks of age (6 weeks corrected age), Estelle is brought to the ED. Her mother is concerned that she is not gaining weight as well as her twin sister, and is 'a miserable baby'.

Estelle's weight is 2.3 kg (below the 0.4th Centile), she looks anxious and thin, and appears mildly jaundiced. There is no organomegaly. The serum total bilirubin is 127 μmol/L.

What is the working diagnosis?

Estelle is reviewed by the Paediatric Registrar, who notes that her nappy appears stained with dark urine, and that she has stools 'the colour of clotted cream'. The registrar is concerned about the possibility of an obstructive jaundice, and takes blood for LFTs, split bilirubin, glucose and clotting. An urgent liver US is arranged.

Results

		Normal
Total bilirubin	130 μmol/L	2–26 μmol/L
Conjugated bilirubin	105 μmol/L	<15% total bilirubin
Albumin	38 g/L	37–50 g/L
Alkaline phosphatase	650 U/L	145–420
ALT	40 U/L	10–40 U/L
Blood glucose	3.0 mmol/L	3.5–7.0 mmol/L
Clotting: normal		

Liver ultrasound (pre-feed) – no gallbladder seen, moderately dilated intrahepatic bile ducts

What should you do next?

An urgent referral is made to the Paediatric liver unit. Further investigations confirm the diagnosis of extrahepatic biliary atresia, and a Kasai portoenterostomy is performed at 14 weeks of age (8 weeks corrected age).

The bilirubin falls, the stools became pigmented, and Estelle begins to gain weight. Her first year is complicated by two episodes of ascending cholangitis, treated rapidly with iv antibiotics. At 4 years of age, Estelle is found to have portal hypertension and evidence of cirrhosis.

Estelle's mother complains, stating that the initial delay in diagnosis caused the Kasai procedure to be delayed

Avoiding Errors in Paediatrics, First Edition. Joseph E. Raine, Kate Williams and Jonathan Bonser.
© 2013 John Wiley & Sons, Ltd. Published 2013 by Blackwell Publishing Ltd.

and the surgical result to be suboptimal, and that this has increased her risk of requiring an early liver transplant.

Expert opinion

Jaundice is common in preterm babies, but in the absence of haemolysis or sepsis usually resolves. Jaundice in a preterm baby persisting for longer than 3 weeks (2 weeks in term infants) is defined as 'prolonged jaundice'. If the conjugated bilirubin fraction is ≥20 μmol/L and >20% of the total bilirubin then investigations for possible liver disease should be instigated urgently.

Skin pigmentation can impair the clinical assessment of jaundice, but dark urine and pale stools are cardinal signs of biliary obstruction, for which a cause must be found promptly. These signs were not asked about by the GP. Biliary atresia can present with a total bilirubin well below the phototherapy threshold, as seen in Estelle.

Vomiting is a relatively common neonatal symptom, but failure to gain weight, particularly in a preterm baby, requires investigation and this sign should have been taken more seriously. Infants who are failing to thrive should be followed up assiduously.

The outcome of surgical treatment of Biliary Atresia is related to the age at surgery, with the best outcomes in those operated on before 30 days of age, although the majority of patients with Biliary Atresia will eventually require liver transplantation.

Legal comment

The hospital's decision to discharge Estelle at 10 days of age when she was minimally jaundiced but gaining weight does not seem to attract the criticism of the expert. The chief criticism is reserved for the GP who saw Estelle at 3 weeks of age, when she was suffering from 'prolonged jaundice'. The GP failed to ask relevant questions about the urine and stools and failed to investigate the jaundice.

The result of these failures was that the biliary atresia was not investigated for another nine weeks, and not treated for two weeks after that. The outcome is said to have been 'suboptimal'.

The hospital can deny all liability in this case. The GP's lawyers (who will be appointed by her MDO) will investigate the probable outcome of an earlier Kasai portoenterostomy, and will negotiate a settlement based on the extent to which the baby's future pain and suffering might have been avoided. However, since the majority of patients with this diagnosis do go on to need a liver transplant, the GP will probably not have to compensate Estelle for *all* her future pain and suffering.

Key learning points

Specific to the case

1. Visual assessment of jaundice lacks accuracy, especially in infants with pigmented skin.
2. Failure to thrive has a wide differential diagnosis.
3. Always exclude conjugated hyperbilirubinemia in infants with prolonged jaundice.
4. The outcome of initial surgery for Biliary Atresia is time dependent.

General points

1. Beware of jumping to premature conclusions on the basis of common symptoms.

Further reading and references

British Society of Paediatric Gastroenterology, Hepatology and Nutrition (2007) Investigation of Neonatal Conjugated Hyperbilirubinaemia. http://www.bspghan.org.uk

Serinet, M-O et al. (2009) Impact of age at Kasai operation on its results in late childhood and adolescence: a rational basis for biliary atresia screening. *Pediatrics* 123: 1280.

Yellow Alert Jaundice Campaign (2011) http://www.yellowalert.org

Case 11 A child with leukaemia and tummy ache

Simon, a 4-year-old boy with Acute Lymphoblastic Leukaemia (ALL), has just completed his second delayed intensification in the current UK ALL trial at the regional Paediatric Oncology Centre (POC). His parents phone the children's ward at the local DGH, their Paediatric Oncology Shared Care Unit (POSCU), to which they have open access. Simon is complaining of tummy ache and has had two episodes of loose stools containing a small amount of blood. His parents have taken his temperature and it is 38.7°C. The nurses have advised them to come in for review and on arrival his temperature is 37.4°C, pulse 140/min, BP 120/50 mmHg and respiratory rate 40/minute. He is seen within 10 minutes by Dr Joseph, the ST1 doctor, who learns that before Simon's recent chemotherapy he had had intermittent abdominal pain and minor bleeding opening his bowels due to constipation, a common problem during treatment with vincristine. Regular lactulose is helping. His younger sister also had tummy ache and loose stools a few days ago and is now well. On examination, Simon is cheerful and cooperative and is well-perfused with warm hands and feet. His chest is clear, heart sounds are normal and his central line site appears clean. His abdomen is slightly distended but soft with possibly some right lower quadrant tenderness but no guarding and normal bowel sounds. The anus is slightly red with a small tear to which Dr Joseph ascribes the recent bleeding. His buccal mucosa is inflamed with some sloughing. Simon's shared care record shows that on discharge from the POC two days previously the haemoglobin was 11.9 g/dL (normal 12–15 g/dL) and the WCC was 4.5×10^9/L (4.5–13×10^9/L) with neutrophils of 3.1×10^9/L (1.5–6×10^9). Dr Joseph consults the POC sepsis guidelines and decides that because the temperature is now below the threshold for treatment, and as Simon is unlikely to be neutropenic yet following his recent chemotherapy, he does not need immediate antibiotics. Dr Joseph makes a diagnosis of probable viral gastroenteritis but asks the nurses to send all his bloods including blood cultures and advises that she will review the results as soon as they are available. Simon is admitted for observation.

Do you agree with this management plan? Would you have done anything differently?

Thirty minutes later Dr Joseph is bleeped and told that the central line will not sample. She gives a verbal instruction to start a 4 hour urokinase infusion and to put some local anaesthetic cream on a few peripheral veins. Dr Joseph returns 2 hours later and is surprised but pleased to insert a cannula easily despite the multiple drips that Simon has had prior to his central line. He is extremely cooperative and has warm hands with easily visible veins.

What would be your assessment of this scenario?

One hour later the nurses call to say that Simon is very quiet and sleepy. His temperature is 38.8°C, pulse 190/min and they cannot measure his BP. They have commenced oxygen treatment because his saturations in air were 78%. On examination Simon is obtunded, has a central capillary refill time of 3 secs, warm peripheries and a respiratory rate of 60/min. A capillary lactate is 7.4 mmol/L (normal<2 mmol/L). The ST4 is called and makes a diagnosis of Gram negative shock, gives 2 boluses of 0.9% saline and calls the anaesthetist. Simon is intubated, ventilated and commenced on inotropes. He is transferred to the PICU at the POC but sadly dies 4 days later of multiorgan failure. His parents file a law suit based on the failure to recognize his illness on admission, the failure to follow available guidelines and the resulting delay in starting treatment culminating in his death. They quote the fact that ALL has an overall 5-year survival rate of 85%.

Avoiding Errors in Paediatrics, First Edition. Joseph E. Raine, Kate Williams and Jonathan Bonser.
© 2013 John Wiley & Sons, Ltd. Published 2013 by Blackwell Publishing Ltd.

Expert opinion

Febrile neutropenia is a medical emergency in children receiving chemotherapy due to the risk of Gram negative sepsis in an immunocompromised host which has an estimated mortality of 40–50%. Once cancer is in remission, infection is the commonest cause of death. The risk is highest following intensive chemotherapy courses but can occur at any time during treatment. All POCs have guidelines for the management of fever in a child undergoing chemotherapy which include temperature thresholds for urgent treatment (often 1 temperature of 38.5°C or 2 temperatures of 38°C in a 4 hour period) plus the advice that any unwell child should receive immediate antibiotics (usually within 1 hour) irrespective of the temperature and the recent neutrophil count. Simon's almost normal temperature on admission was irrelevant because the parents had already documented a fever that exceeded the threshold for treatment. Knowing this they may have already given paracetamol at home, a point that was not asked about by Dr Joseph. Neutrophil counts can drop very quickly especially with an intercurrent illness and treatment must not be delayed by waiting for results.

Simon's temperature at home was sufficiently high to merit urgent broad spectrum iv antibiotics but he also had evidence of physiological compromise on admission. He was tachypneic, had a tachycardia that was not explicable by either fever or anaemia and had a wide pulse pressure. As in this case, children and young adults can maintain or even raise their systolic blood pressure until late in shock. Hypotension indicates critical illness and impending death. Simon has mouth and abdominal signs consistent with chemotherapy induced mucositis/typhilitis (neutropaenic caecal inflammation), as well as appendicitis putting him at high risk of the transmural passage of Gram negative organisms and the resulting characteristic shock. This risk should have been detected on admission and certainly when the cannula was inserted so easily. Cooperative 4 year olds with cannulas are very unusual. It is likely that prompt treatment would have saved Simon's life.

 Legal comment

It is probable that earlier treatment would have averted Simon's death. That in itself would mean that compensation would be payable. The parents do not need to quote 5 year survival figures. It is enough to show that Simon would have survived this particular episode. Compensation, however, will be limited to a statutory sum of £11,800 for bereavement damages, the cost of Simon's funeral and a sum for the pain and suffering that he endured in the days leading up to his death.

There appear to have been a number of mistakes in Simon's treatment, as detailed in the Expert Opinion. Dr Joseph had read the POC guidelines, but had misinterpreted them. The parents had reported a high temperature at home and that should have been enough to trigger the administration of antibiotics. Perhaps the guidelines were not clear, in which case someone should try to improve them. That would be a systems failure.

Dr Joseph was on the right tracks. She at least looked at the guidelines. However, she should probably have recognized that this could be a complicated case and contacted someone with more experience to review the child.

 Key learning points

Specific to the case
1. Fever in an immunocompromised patient is an emergency. It is safest to err on the side of caution and to start antibiotics immediately pending blood and culture results.
2. Always clarify the prehospital management and ensure that observations are not just documented but interpreted appropriately.
3. Beware of 'warm shock'.

General points
1. Tachycardia with no obvious cause should never be ignored and can be due to severe sepsis.
2. Hypotension is a late sign in shocked children and young adults and indicates critical illness and impending death.
3. Always read available guidelines thoroughly before making a decision and if in doubt seek senior advice including that from experienced nurses.
4. Be 'suspicious' of young children who are cooperative with painful procedures.

Further reading and references

Read your regional oncology units shared care protocols.
Schwartz AJ (2011) *Shock in Pediatrics.* http://emedicine.medscape.com/article/1833578-overview

Case 12 A boy with fever and rigors

Sanjay, a previously healthy 7-year-old boy, presents to the ED with a 3-day history of fever and rigors. He had been seen by his GP and diagnosed with influenza 2 days earlier, and was advised to take antipyretics. Sanjay looks unwell but there are no abnormal findings on examination apart from a temperature of 38.4°C and heart rate of 115/minute. Urinalysis is unremarkable. The ED doctor decides to take some bloods which show a WCC of 16.3 × 10⁹/L (normal 4.5–13 × 10⁹/L), neutrophils 11.3 × 10⁹/L (2–6 × 10⁹/L) and a CRP of 99 mg/L (<6 mg/L). He refers Sanjay to the Paediatric ST2 for a second opinion as he has no focus for the fever.

How would you manage the child at this point?

A second physical examination confirms that there is no obvious focus of infection. Sanjay is admitted to the Paediatric ward with a provisional diagnosis of sepsis. A CXR is done and urine and blood cultures are taken. He is commenced on iv ceftriaxone at a dose of 50 mg/kg. He has one more spike of fever (38.8°C) overnight, but by the next morning he is feeling a little better. On the ward round the registrar decides to continue the antibiotics for 48 hours pending the blood culture results. Late in the afternoon the ST2 receives a telephone call from the microbiology registrar to inform him that the blood cultures are growing Staphylococci, and he advises that treatment be continued until further results are available. The next day Sanjay is feeling much better and has been afebrile for 12 hours. Thorough physical examination remains unremarkable. The organism isolated from the blood culture is confirmed as *Staphylococcus aureus* and the microbiologist recommends changing treatment to iv flucloxacillin. However, the Paediatric team elects to continue with once daily ceftriaxone so that Sanjay can receive ambulatory treatment for a total of one week.

What do you think of this management strategy?

Two weeks later Sanjay returns to the ED in the evening, with increasing malaise and a low-grade fever over the last 5 days. He now has a 2/6 ejection systolic murmur loudest in the aortic area and an early diastolic murmur, and has 2+ blood and 1+ protein on urine dipstick analysis.

What is the likely diagnosis and what would you do now?

Sanjay is readmitted to the paediatric ward and after blood cultures have been taken he is commenced on intravenous ceftriaxone again. During the night he is found collapsed on the floor of the ward toilet, unresponsive. He is subsequently found to have had an embolic stroke as a result of vegetations on a previously undiagnosed bicuspid aortic valve. Although Sanjay survives, he has persistent neurological deficits that affect his speech and movement, and frequent seizures. His parents sue the hospital claiming that the diagnosis of infective endocarditis was completely missed and that this caused their son to have an adverse outcome.

Expert opinion

Staphylococcus aureus bacteraemia is frequently associated with a focus of infection: this may be an abscess or an infected prosthetic or intravascular device, and it is an increasingly common cause of endocarditis. The source of the infection should be actively sought, and removed if feasible. Recommended investigations include a CXR, abdominal US and echocardiography. Flucloxacillin is the preferred antibiotic in most cases, and the usual duration of iv antibiotic therapy is at least 14 days for uncomplicated infections with no focus of infection (or following removal of a focus) and 4–6

Avoiding Errors in Paediatrics, First Edition. Joseph E. Raine, Kate Williams and Jonathan Bonser.
© 2013 John Wiley & Sons, Ltd. Published 2013 by Blackwell Publishing Ltd.

weeks when there is a deep focus of infection such as osteomyelitis. In this case the reason for the *S. aureus* bacteremia in Sanjay was not adequately investigated, the duration of treatment was less than recommended, and the decision to use once daily ceftriaxone instead of flucloxacillin may have reduced the effectiveness of treatment. Sanjay probably had infective endocarditis at the time of the initial presentation, and even if vegetations were not visible at that time, the presence of a valvular abnormality would have increased the index of suspicion. Absence of a murmur on physical examination does not exclude infective endocarditis, and failure to investigate adequately with an echocardiogram after finding *S. aureus* in the blood cultures is highly likely to have contributed to the subsequent adverse events.

 Legal comment

It seems that an expert will say that the failure to look for a focus of infection after *Staphylococcus aureus* had been identified and to then treat it properly could not be justified by any responsible body of medical opinion.

The hospital will therefore be responsible for all the consequences of that failure. The hospital's lawyers may wish to explore whether, by the time *Staphylococcus aureus* was identified, it was too late for iv flucloxacillin to have prevented the stroke. But that may be a forlorn hope.

Failing that, this case is going to be very expensive for the Trust as Sanjay is very young and is going to need a lot of care all his life. He and his parents can expect compensation for the cost of his care for his whole life, and for his pain and suffering.

Compensation for the cost of care will be calculated by evaluating the cost of Sanjay's needs for a year and then applying a multiplier to reflect his expected longevity. Depending on the strength of the case and Sanjay's life expectancy, any settlement is likely to be well over a million pounds and could easily be several million pounds.

 Key learning points

Specific to the case

1. In any patient with a serious (including bacteraemia) or unusual bacterial infection you should ask: why has this patient got this infection at this time?

2. Patients with *S. aureus* bacteraemia should have an echocardiogram as part of the routine assessment looking for a focus of infection.
3. The most appropriate antibiotic and duration of treatment of *S. aureus* bacteraemia should be decided in consultation with a microbiologist or infectious diseases specialist.
4. A bicuspid aortic valve is the most common congenital cardiac abnormality, present in 1–2% of individuals, and it is frequently undetectable on routine clinical examination. Despite this it is a significant risk factor for infective endocarditis.
5. Left-sided valvular endocarditis can result in systemic (including cerebral) septic emboli, leading to metastatic sites of infection and vascular occlusion.

General points

1. Not all congenital cardiac defects are easily detected at birth, and some may remain asymptomatic throughout childhood.
2. Infective endocarditis can occur on both abnormal and normal heart valves, with central venous catheters being a significant risk factor in the latter case.
3. *S. aureus* bacteraemia is a frequent complication of intravascular devices, which should be promptly removed.
4. Although once daily antibiotic treatment regimes are convenient and allow management of patients on an ambulatory basis, they should only be used when they are as effective as other treatment regimens.

Further reading and references

Day MD *et al.* (2009) Characteristics of children hospitalized with infective endocarditis. *Circulation* 119(6): 865–70.

Thwaites GE *et al.* (2011) Clinical management of Staphylococcus aureus bacteraemia. *Lancet Infect Dis* 11(3): 208–22.

Sharland M (ed.) (2011) *Manual of Childhood Infections*, 3rd edn. Oxford: Oxford University Press.

Valente AM *et al.* (2005) Frequency of infective endocarditis among infants and children with Staphylococcus aureus bacteremia. *Pediatrics* 115(1): e15–19.

Case 13 A stiff hand

A male infant, Rory, was born at 39 weeks gestation, weighing 3.92 kg. His mother developed chickenpox 3 days prior to his birth.

What are the implications for the baby?

Rory was in good condition at birth, but in view of the maternal history, he was treated with intramuscular varicella-zoster immune globulin (ZIG), and a decision was made to treat him with prophylactic iv aciclovir, 10 mg/kg 8 hourly for 7 days. An iv cannula was sited in the dorsum of the left hand with some difficulty, and aciclovir was commenced by iv infusion.

Shortly after commencement of the second dose of aciclovir, the nurse thought that Rory seemed unsettled, stopped the infusion, and called the neonatal ST3 to review him. The doctor examined the infant and thought he appeared well, the iv line flushed easily when tested with a bolus of 0.9% sodium chloride, and no abnormal signs were noted. The infusion was continued.

Half way through the third dose of aciclovir, Rory appeared to be in pain, and the infusion was stopped. The ST3 reviewed Rory, and found his left hand to be swollen and tense, with a white area 2 × 1.5 cm in diameter over the dorsum of the hand.

What would you do next? What physical signs are important?

The ST3 removed the cannula and called his registrar for help. On review, 30 minutes later, the fingers had normal perfusion, the radial and ulnar pulses were normal, but the dorsum of the hand and wrist were very swollen and tense, with a white mottled area on the dorsum of the hand as described previously.

After referring to the hospital's extravasation policy, the subcutaneous tissue of the dorsum of the hand was thoroughly irrigated with 0.9% sodium chloride, wide bore needle holes were made in the skin peripheral to the

pale area, and saline solution injected into the pale area. The perfusion of the dorsum of the hand appeared to improve. The hand was dressed and elevated. Aciclovir was continued via a new cannula in a larger and more proximal vein.

What follow-up is needed?

By 24 hours, an ulcer had developed at the site of the cannula, measuring 4 × 6 mm. The ulcer healed slowly by epithelialization from the periphery of the ulcer, and left a scar on the dorsum of the hand measuring 4 mm in diameter.

Rory did not develop chickenpox, and was discharged home at the age of 10 days.

At six months of age, Rory's parents complained that their son had difficulty extending his left middle and ring fingers. A plastic surgeon was consulted, who found scarring and tethering of the extensor tendons of the left middle and ring fingers. Rory's parents made a complaint stating that the iv aciclovir infusion had been inadequately monitored and that this had led to all the subsequent problems.

 Expert opinion

Maternal chickenpox at the end of pregnancy carries a risk of transmission of the virus to the fetus, which may result in severe haemorrhagic neonatal chickenpox. Rory's mother is infectious to the fetus when she is viraemic, and thus can infect her baby whilst incubating her infection, even if her symptoms develop postnatally. As she has not had time to mount an immune response to the virus, if maternal symptoms occur from seven days before delivery to seven days postnatally, the baby will have no passive immunity to chickenpox, and should receive passive immunization with ZIG. Intravenous aciclovir should also be considered for infants whose mothers develop chickenpox four days before to

---

Avoiding Errors in Paediatrics, First Edition. Joseph E. Raine, Kate Williams and Jonathan Bonser.
© 2013 John Wiley & Sons, Ltd. Published 2013 by Blackwell Publishing Ltd.

two days after delivery as they are at the highest risk of a fatal outcome despite ZIG prophylaxis.

Aciclovir is an irritant drug when made up as an iv infusion, with an alkaline pH of 11. It is wise to give such infusions into large veins or to use a central line, so that the infusion is rapidly diluted by the blood within the vein flowing past the cannula tip. It is particularly important that the iv line is closely observed, that the infusion site is monitored, and that action is taken immediately if there is a suspicion that the line is not working. Very young children are at increased risk of extravasation, because their tissues are more delicate, and they are less able to communicate.

In this case, line insertion was difficult (possibly traumatizing the lining of the vein), and a relatively small vein was used. The nurse noticed irritability (possibly indicating pain), and it would have been prudent to re-site the cannula even though the initial insertion had been difficult.

The appearance of the iv site after the extravasation suggests that a significant volume of the infusate had entered the soft tissues, raising questions about the vigilance of monitoring of the infusion site.

Once the extravasation had been identified, the infusion should have been stopped, but the cannula should not have been removed until an attempt had been made to aspirate as much of the drug as possible through the cannula.

Flushing of the soft tissues with 0.9% saline was a reasonable emergency response to this injury, but an early consultation with a plastic surgeon would have been wise, particularly once evidence of ulceration had been seen.

Careful follow-up of the hand and physiotherapy to maintain a physiological range of movement of the wrist and fingers might have reduced the subsequent disability.

 Legal comment

The parents have complained to the hospital about the treatment that their child has received. Although it was wise to administer aciclovir to Rory, a number of mistakes were made in the administration of the aciclovir and then in the aftercare, as detailed in the Expert Opinion, and the hospital should apologize immediately. It will be easy for the parents to prove that the treatment was negligent and if they pursue a claim it will be successful. But Rory is only a baby and it will be some time before it becomes clear how the tethering of the tendons has affected him and a lawyer instructed by the family would probably wish to wait a few years to see how the condition develops, before pressing for compensation. After all, Rory will have until he is 21 to bring a claim. The affected hand is the left hand and it may not be the dominant hand, but the disability may prevent him from taking a job that requires manual dexterity. The value of the claim will probably be low: between £5000 and £20,000. However, if the injury is found to limit his earning capacity, then the damages will be increased accordingly.

 Key learning points

Specific to the case
1. Aciclovir infusions are irritant and strongly alkaline, use a big vein or a central line whenever possible.
2. Read the Summary of Product Characteristics of drugs that you prescribe.
3. Pay attention to nursing concerns about the behaviour of children for whom they are caring – early signs are often subtle.
4. Make a clear follow up plan for children who experience complications of treatment.
5. Obtain expert advice promptly.

General points
1. Communicate with parents clearly and honestly when a child experiences a treatment related complication.
2. Adverse outcomes to prophylactic interventions are highly distressing to parents.

Further reading and references

Health Protection Agency (2011) Guidance on Viral Rash in Pregnancy. www.hpa.org.uk.

eMC (2011) Summary of Product Characteristics, Aciclovir 250mg Powder for Solution for Infusion, www.medicines.org.uk

British National Formulary (2011) Extravasation. bnfc.org/bnfc/bnfc/current/100049.htm

Case 14 A serious feeding problem

Tanya is born at 18.30, at 41 weeks gestation following a normal pregnancy. She has Apgar scores of 8 at 1 minute and 9 at 5 minutes and weighs 3.12 kg. Tanya's mother received an epidural for pain relief, and labour lasted for 15 hours. Tanya looks well, and is put to the breast in the labour ward.

During the evening, Tanya's mother feels hot and shivery and is reviewed by the Obstetric ST3, who thinks that the cause might be a urinary tract infection, sends a maternal urine sample to the laboratory, and prescribes amoxicillin.

What are the implications of this finding for the baby?

The following morning at 06.10, it is noted that Tanya has stopped latching onto the breast. She requires supplementary feeding using expressed breast milk by nasogastric tube, and is put to the breast every 3 hours. At 14.30, the midwife notices that Tanya is grunting and tachypnoeic, and calls the neonatal ST2 to examine her. The ST2 reviews Tanya at 14.45, and observes that she is grunting and pale, with a respiratory rate of 90/min, and a heart rate of 180/min. Her CRT is 2 secs. She is admitted to NICU immediately.

What information do you need?

On admission to NICU, Tanya's temperature is 36°C, her pulse 185/min, and her blood pressure 88/50 mmHg. Her respiratory rate is 100/min with recession and expiratory grunting. Her oxygen saturation is 82% in air, rising to 93% in 50% oxygen. Her capillary blood gas shows a pH 7.15 (normal 7.35–7.45), PCO_2 8.4 kPa (4.7–6.4 kPa) and lactate 6.0 mmol/L (<2mmol/L).

What further tests should you do?

An iv line is sited, and blood cultures are taken. A FBC is sent, and a CXR is requested. The blood glu-

cose is 8.4 mmol/L (2.8–4.5 mmol/L). Intravenous benzylpenicillin and gentamicin are administered at 15.05. Shortly afterwards, the FBC is reported: Hb 17.4 g/dL (14–22 g/dL), WBC 6.2 × 10⁹/L (9–30 × 10⁹/L), neutrophils 0.5 × 10⁹/L (4–24 × 10⁹/L), platelets 65 × 10⁹/L (150–400 × 10⁹/L). Tanya's CXR shows widespread patchy consolidation, with a small pleural effusion at the left base. Shortly after the CXR, Tanya starts to have profound apnoeas and requires intermittent positive pressure ventilation.

What is your working diagnosis?

At 17.00 the microbiology laboratory reports that the mother's urine has a heavy growth of a Gram positive coccus. Tanya continues to deteriorate, becomes oliguric and hypotensive, and requires inotropic support with dopamine and noradrenaline infusions for 2 days. She is ventilated for 6 days, and receives iv benzylenicillin and gentamicin for 10 days. A lumbar puncture is done and the CSF is sterile, but her blood cultures produce a heavy growth of Group B beta haemolytic streptococcus. At follow-up, she is developmentally delayed with acquired microcephaly.

Tanya's mother makes a complaint stating that her daughter's developmental delay resulted from delayed treatment of her septicaemia.

Expert opinion

Early-onset Group B Streptococcal (GBS) Septicaemia has a fulminant presentation. Although the labour went well, and this appeared to be a low risk delivery, the mother's symptoms immediately postnatally suggest that she is likely to have had a Group B streptococcal urinary tract infection in labour that was undiagnosed. A maternal GBS urinary tract infection is a marker of heavy maternal colonization, and increases the risk of neonatal infection approximately 10-fold.

If the maternal infection had been recognized antenatally, the mother would have been offered

Avoiding Errors in Paediatrics, First Edition. Joseph E. Raine, Kate Williams and Jonathan Bonser.
© 2013 John Wiley & Sons, Ltd. Published 2013 by Blackwell Publishing Ltd.

intrapartum penicillin prophylaxis, to reduce the risk of vertical transmission of the infection. In the UK, there is currently (2011) no national screening programme for GBS in pregnancy, although GBS screening in late pregnancy is routine in the USA, because the prevalence of maternal GBS carriage is significantly higher there than in the UK.

Postnatal antibiotic prophylaxis for the infant of a GBS colonized mother has been shown to be ineffective, but vigilance for symptoms and early treatment of the symptomatic baby is essential.

In this case, there was no postnatal communication between the obstetric and neonatal teams. The mother was managed independently, and the implications of her infection for Tanya were not considered.

Failure of a term baby to feed requires active investigation – any term baby who needs a nasogastric tube requires a formal diagnosis. In this case, it is highly likely that the feeding difficulties were due to the combination of tachypnoea and floppiness, resulting from bacterial sepsis.

It is thus clear that there was at least an eight-hour delay in initiating treatment, and that if more intensive observation of the baby had been instituted when her mother had a rigor, it is distinctly possible that Tanya may have been treated earlier and that the neurological sequelae could have been avoided.

The microcephaly that was subsequently identified was a consequence of injury to the white matter of the brain as a result of the septic shock.

 Legal comment

Tanya's mother has complained to the hospital about the treatment of her newborn baby. If she seeks compensation, then this could be a £1,000,000+ claim at full valuation, depending on the severity of the developmental delay and its future implications for Tanya's life. The extent of the claim will depend on the answers to such questions as: will Tanya be able to find employment and will she need a carer when she reaches maturity?

We say 'full valuation', because there could be significant question marks concerning causation. Treatment should probably have been started earlier, but initially, Tanya is likely to have just been observed. The real question is: when would a reasonable doctor have started intensive antibiotic treatment? It is likely that the opinions of the instructed experts will differ. Clearly the hypothetical time when Tanya 'should' have received treatment may make a difference to whether her microcephaly and developmental delay could have been avoided.

It is, therefore, likely that any claim will be settled at a discount.

The main error here appears to be a systems failure: the mother's postnatal infection was not communicated to the paediatric team. The Obstetric and Paediatric Departments need to talk to each other!

 Key learning points

Specific to the case

1. Sepsis in neonates may be of very rapid onset.
2. Maternal sepsis may have serious implications for neonates, even if the symptoms present postnatally.
3. Septic neonates may be afebrile or hypothermic.
4. When a mature baby needs a tube feed, search vigorously for an underlying cause.

General points

1. Timely communication between Midwifery, Obstetric and Neonatal teams underpins safe management of both mother and baby.

Further reading and references

Group B Streptococcus Support. www.gbss.org.uk

Royal College of Obstetricians and Gynaecologists (2003) Prevention of Early Onset Neonatal Group B Streptococcal Disease: Green Top 36. www.rcog.org.uk

Case 15 Fits, faints and funny turns

A 15-year-old girl called Nina is referred to outpatients with a 2-year history of abnormal episodes. The GP originally diagnosed them as being vasovagal but she is seeking advice because they have changed recently. The consultant general paediatrician documents the history from Nina and her mother. Nina says some are predictable and occur when she stands up too quickly and this can make her feel hot, sweaty and dizzy. The next thing she remembers is waking up on the floor with staff or friends expressing concern. She recovers after about 10 minutes. She had a minor head injury during one episode. Her mother describes her as 'ghostly white' and states that she has had occasional, brief (10 seconds), symmetrical shaking of all 4 limbs. However, in the past 6 months Nina has had at least 12 new episodes that her family have never witnessed. She has no warning, but school staff and friends say that she stiffens all over, loses awareness and 'drops to the floor like a rag doll'. Sometimes she has jerking movements of her legs. There is no colour change. She has bitten the tip of her tongue twice but there has been no other injury and no incontinence. She is back to normal within minutes.

Nina is making good progress in Year 10 and has a stable group of friends. She has missed some school and has been banned from sport because of these episodes. Apart from menorrhagia and irregular periods there is no other history of note. Examination is normal including fundoscopy and lying and standing blood pressures.

Does she have epilepsy?

The consultant agrees that the first episodes were vasovagal but is concerned that the new episodes are seizures. An ECG, EEG and MRI scan are normal. He asks the family to keep a diary, and at review 6 weeks later there have been another 8 events, all either at school or when out with her friends. He makes a diagnosis of epilepsy, prescribes sodium valproate 1g bd and makes an appointment for 6 months.

Was this reasonable management?

At the next appointment Nina's family report severe drowsiness at the start of treatment with 3 further weeks off school. The frequency and pattern of the episodes is unchanged. The consultant concludes that these are myoclonic seizures and adds clonazepam. Nina reports that her periods have become even more irregular and that she has not had a bleed for 4 months. She denies being sexually active. The consultant explains that sodium valproate can cause menstrual irregularity due to the polycystic ovary syndrome.

What would you have done?

Six months later Nina returns to clinic with her parents and her 6-week-old baby boy. He has significant congenital abnormalities – Tetralogy of Fallot, cleft palate and hypospadias – picked up on a late antenatal scan at 29 weeks gestation when she realized she was pregnant. Nina stopped both drugs immediately and has had no episodes since.

The family file a lawsuit claiming that the consultant was not an expert in epilepsy and should not have treated their daughter. In particular, they complain that Nina should have been warned about the potential teratogenic effects of sodium valproate despite her denial (in front of her mother) of being sexually active.

Expert opinion

A diagnosis of epilepsy is a life-altering event for any patient and family. It is made primarily from the history. Fits, faints, jerks and blackouts are common in children but almost half of those referred to a tertiary paediatric neurologist with a suggested diagnosis of epilepsy do not have the condition. It is crucial to get it right but it is often difficult. An EEG can support the clinical diagnosis, determine the seizure type and help with

Avoiding Errors in Paediatrics, First Edition. Joseph E. Raine, Kate Williams and Jonathan Bonser.
© 2013 John Wiley & Sons, Ltd. Published 2013 by Blackwell Publishing Ltd.

treatment. A MRI scan may identify structural abnormalities that cause certain, usually focal, epilepsies. Neither diagnose epilepsy. Nina's first episodes were clearly vasovagal but the second episodes were almost certainly pseudo-seizures, not an uncommon diagnosis in teenage girls. Particular pointers are that, despite their frequency, they had never been witnessed by the family, the lack of injuries and biting the tip of the tongue – patients are aware that people often 'bite their tongue' during a fit, but do not realise that it is never the tip.

There are comprehensive NICE guidelines for the management of epilepsy in children and young people with one of the key recommendations being that all children with a recent-onset suspected seizure should be seen urgently by a specialist. The latter was defined as 'a paediatrician with training and expertise in the epilepsies'. The British Paediatric Neurology Association has developed Paediatric Epilepsy Training (PET) courses and it would now be considered bad practice for a child to be managed by a doctor in secondary care who has not completed at least a PET 1 course. Making the diagnosis is rarely urgent and it is more important to obtain witnessed accounts and video evidence and to refer to a tertiary neurologist if there is continued doubt. Having made the wrong diagnosis, the doctor compounded his errors by incurring severe side effects with a huge initial dose of valproate which lead to significant sedation, delaying a review for 6 months and then using polypharmacy instead of following the principles of monotherapy. There was no involvement of an Epilepsy Specialist Nurse and the doctor failed to counsel Nina who is of child-bearing age. Despite her public denial, the risk of her being sexually active was significant and there should have been a confidential discussion to ensure that she understood the risks of sodium valproate and the need to plan a pregnancy. All staff dealing with children with chronic diseases must have disease-specific and generic skills to manage and communicate with adolescents. This doctor failed to recognize their limitations and that they were practising outside their field of expertise.

 Legal comment

This could be a complicated legal case. Nina may be able to make a claim for what could be termed an unwanted pregnancy (in the sense that she may have sought a termination, if the pregnancy had been diagnosed sufficiently early and the foetus' abnormalities had been explained to her).

However, the claim of Nina, the mother of the baby, is academic. The fact is that the paediatrican should have referred Nina to a paediatric neurologist or to a paediatrician with a special interest in epilepsy; his failure to do this amounts to a breach of duty. If he had done this, then Nina would not have been diagnosed as suffering from epilepsy and the sodium valproate would not have been prescribed. It is likely that an instructed expert will conclude that her baby's abnormalities were caused by the sodium valproate.

On this analysis, the baby will have a valid claim against the hospital in his own right; he was damaged in utero by the negligence of the doctor. Experts will need to examine the baby to judge the extent of his disabilities and how they will affect him in his future life. The claim could be worth several hundred thousand pounds, especially if the instructed experts conclude that the baby suffers from developmental delay as a result of the sodium valproate.

 Key learning points

Specific to the case

1. Fits, faints, jerks and blackouts are common in children but less than half of these will be epileptic seizures.
2. Making a diagnosis of epilepsy is rarely urgent but it is crucial to get it right.
3. All children with epilepsy should be managed by a paediatrician with specific training and expertise.

General points

1. One fundamental skill required of all doctors at all levels is to recognize the limits of their experience and expertise. There is no shame in doing so and in asking for help.
2. All staff caring for adolescents need to have the skills to manage this age group and to communicate effectively with them.

Further reading and references

NICE (2012) Epilepsy: NICE Guideline. http://guidance.nice.org.uk/CG137/NICEGuidance/pdf/English

SIGN (Scottish Intercollegiate Guidelines Network) (2005) Diagnosis and Management of Epilepsies in Children and Young People: A National Clinical Guideline. www.sign.ac.uk/pdf/sign81.pdf

Case 16 A hospital acquired infection

Charlie, a 7-week-old male infant who was born at 24 weeks gestation, is transferred from the regional level 3 neonatal unit back to the intermediate care neonatal nursery at the hospital of birth. He remains oxygen dependent and on intermittent CPAP, is enterally fed via a nasogastric tube, and is receiving medical therapy for gastro-oesophageal reflux. Charlie had bilateral grade 2 intraventricular haemorrhages, and his parents are anxious about his long-term prognosis. Charlie's parents are also worried about the transfer back to the local hospital, because they felt that the care they received at the time of delivery was not optimal.

What actions should be routinely taken when a baby is transferred to a neonatal unit from another hospital?

Charlie's parents are also anxious about the fact that there is a baby with Methicillin Resistant *Staphylococcus aureus* (MRSA) colonization in a side-room adjacent to their son's incubator. They have heard about MRSA and are worried that it might spread to Charlie.

What should the parents be told about MRSA?

On the third day after arrival Charlie has a profound apnoeic episode during a feed. Due to a staffing shortage there is only one nurse in the intermediate nursery who is relatively inexperienced but she immediately calls the doctor for help. The ST2 doctor is in the side-room with the MRSA-colonized baby, and runs straight out to assist the nurse without removing his apron and gloves. Charlie is now bradycardic and requires mask ventilation for a minute before starting to recover. Charlie's parents watch the whole event and are clearly terrified.

What else would you do at this stage?

Unfortunately, 2 weeks later, Charlie has another profound apnoeic episode during feeding and requires intubation and ventilation for presumed aspiration pneumonia. Charlie is transferred back to the regional neonatal intensive care unit, where a scanty growth of MRSA is isolated from the tracheal secretions on one occasion, and antibiotic therapy is adjusted to treat MRSA pneumonia. He has a prolonged period of ventilation, and subsequently has severe chronic lung disease and eventually requires a tracheostomy for subglottic stenosis.

Some months later Charlie's parents approach a lawyer to sue the hospital claiming that their baby acquired MRSA at the local hospital and that this has contributed to his poor outcome. They state that a doctor attended their baby without changing gloves or washing his hands after treating a patient known to be MRSA positive, and that proper infection control procedures were not followed. Although the nursing notes documented that MRSA swabs were sent when Charlie was admitted to the intermediate nursery, these were never processed because the wrong hospital number was on the swabs, and nobody repeated the swabs.

Expert opinion

Globally, MRSA is an increasingly common cause of hospital acquired infection in infants in NICUs and has been associated with increased mortality, morbidity and cost of hospital care. MRSA is usually not only resistant to methicillin/flucloxacillin but also to macrolides, quinolones and clindamycin, making it more difficult to treat. The treatment of choice is usually vancomycin. There is little clear evidence to guide the optimal approach to screening for MRSA in infants in a neonatal unit, or to guide the optimal management of those infants found to be colonized. However, most units will screen new admissions with swabs taken from several

Avoiding Errors in Paediatrics, First Edition. Joseph E. Raine, Kate Williams and Jonathan Bonser.
© 2013 John Wiley & Sons, Ltd. Published 2013 by Blackwell Publishing Ltd.

different anatomical locations and will physically isolate any infants found to be MRSA positive in a separate room, with barrier precautions (gloves and aprons) for any contact with the colonized infant or his/her surroundings because MRSA can be shed into the environment. Although meticulous hygiene standards should always be practised in neonatal units, prevention of transmission of MRSA relies on continuous adherence to these standards. MRSA transmission is often increased by overcrowding or understaffing of the unit, which reduces the likelihood of staff performing optimal hand hygiene. In this case there was a clear failure of basic hygiene standards when the doctor rushed to the emergency without removing a contaminated apron and gloves. It is very unlikely that the time taken to remove gloves and an apron, and apply alcohol hand gel (as a minimum standard of hand hygiene), would have adversely affected the resuscitation efforts. This may have been the cause of MRSA transmission to the infant, but because the admission swabs were not processed it is impossible to know if Charlie was already MRSA colonized. Furthermore, MRSA may not have actually been the cause of the subsequent pneumonia, but because MRSA was isolated from a tracheal aspirate sample, it was prudent to treat as a MRSA pneumonia.

 Legal comment

In this case, there appears to have been a breach of duty when the doctor did not remove his apron and gloves before treating Charlie. However, it may well be impossible for the parents to prove, on the balance of probabilities, that Charlie's subsequent problems were caused by the transmission of MRSA at this incident. He was already in a precarious situation with intraventricular haemorrhages and reflux, and may have developed the aspiration pneumonia and chronic lung disease anyway.

Some detailed analysis by neonatal experts will have to be carried out. Each of them will have to come to a view on the probable chain of events. If the case came to Court, a judge would have to decide which expert's view on the probable cause is the most cogent. Expert evidence may well be that the transmission of MRSA probably *contributed* to rather than caused chronic lung disease. In that case, to assess the amount of compensation payable, a calculation would have to be made based on the proportion of the baby's ultimate disability which is attributable to the MRSA.

Overall, this would be difficult and risky litigation for the parents.

 Key learning points

Specific to the case

1. Screening for MRSA on admission is recommended for high risk and high prevalence environments such as a neonatal intensive care unit.
2. If MRSA swabs are sent on admission, then the results should be checked and recorded as soon as they are available.
3. Hand hygiene is particularly important to prevent the spread of MRSA between infants in neonatal intensive care units.
4. Understaffing is a key factor facilitating MRSA transmission.
5. Emergency situations are common in intensive care units, but all possible efforts to maintain infection control procedures should be made.
6. Provision of easily accessible alcohol hand-rub and hand washing facilities may increase adherence to hand hygiene policies.

General points

1. Identification of an infant infected or colonized with MRSA or another antibiotic resistant organism (such as extended spectrum beta-lactamase (ESBL) producing organisms) should be seen as a sentinel event and should prompt further action to screen other infants and to prevent or manage an outbreak.
2. Measures to reduce MRSA transmission include reinforcement of hand hygiene measures, isolation of colonized infants, cleaning of the environment surrounding colonized infants, and deep cleaning of the whole unit. Screening of staff may also become necessary.
3. MRSA decolonization for infants in neonatal units is possible, but evidence of the risks and benefits is scarce.
4. It is important to consider changing empirical antibiotic regimes to cover MRSA for the treatment of nosocomial infections in MRSA colonized infants or during an outbreak of MRSA.

Further reading and references

Coia JE *et al.* (2006) Joint Working Party of the British Society of Antimicrobial Chemotherapy; Hospital

Infection Society; Infection Control Nurses Association. Guidelines for the control and prevention of meticillin-resistant Staphylococcus aureus (MRSA) in healthcare facilities. *J Hosp Infect* 63 Suppl 1: S1–44.

Gould FK *et al.* (2009) MRSA Working Party of the British Society for Antimicrobial Chemotherapy. Guidelines (2008) for the prophylaxis and treatment of methicillin-resistant Staphylococcus aureus (MRSA) infections in the United Kingdom. *J Antimicrob Chemother* 63(5): 849–61.

Laing IA *et al.* (2009) Controlling an outbreak of MRSA in the neonatal unit: a steep learning curve. *Arch Dis Child Fetal Neonatal* 94(4): F307–10.

Case 17 Recurrent wheeze

Caroline, a $2\frac{1}{2}$-year-old girl, was brought to the Paediatric ED by staff at her nursery because she had suddenly developed a cough and a wheeze. They reported that she had been well all day and was playing quite happily with a doll after lunch. In accordance with Caroline's parents' instructions, nursery staff had given her 4 puffs of salbutamol via a spacer but she had become very upset and had not improved. When her parents arrived in the ED the ST1 obtained a history of previous viral induced wheeze and treated with salbutamol via a spacer with good effect. The wheeze had initially developed after an episode of bronchiolitis at 7 months of age, for which Caroline had been in hospital for 4 days needing nasogastric feeds and oxygen therapy. There was no history of a recent illness and no other significant medical history. Caroline's father had a history of asthma treated with regular inhaled steroids. Neither parent smoked in the house although her father did outside.

Which part of this history should have been explored in greater detail?

On examination Caroline looked generally well and was not distressed. Her temperature was 37.1°C, pulse 88/minute, respiratory rate 28/minute with mild intercostal and subcostal recession. On auscultation there was bilateral expiratory wheeze greater on the right than the left. There was also reduced air entry in the right lower zone posteriorly. Percussion was normal throughout. The remainder of the examination was unremarkable. Her height and weight both plotted on the 25th centile which was appropriate for the family.

Would you have requested a CXR at this stage? If so, why?

A diagnosis was made of probable viral induced wheeze and the reduced air entry ascribed to probable mucus plugging and atelectasis. She was given 10 puffs of salbutamol via a spacer and when reviewed by the ST5 an hour later her chest was much improved, although there was still some wheeze and the signs at the right base were unchanged. Caroline was discharged home with advice to continue with regular salbutamol for 48 hours or until better. There was a discussion about the possibility that this was a first episode of asthma and that Caroline might in due course require preventative treatment like her father. This was mentioned in the discharge summary to the GP. Her inhaler technique was assessed as adequate.

What is your view of this management?

Three months later Caroline presents again to the ED with a high fever, cough and a wheeze. The ST2 records that she is toxic and flushed with a temperature of 38.7°C, pulse 110/minute, respiratory rate 36/minute and oxygen saturation 92% in air. Auscultation shows widespread wheeze and reduced air entry and dullness at the right base with some crackles. The GP referral letter comments that this is Caroline's third episode in six weeks of right sided signs requiring antibiotics and a CXR he requested during the second episode had shown right lower lobe abnormalities. She is given a salbutamol nebulizer and a dose of paracetamol. A second CXR is requested. An hour later she is reviewed by the ST4. Her temperature is 37.4°C and she is playing in the playroom. He notes her fruity cough and confirms the findings of some dullness and crackles in the right base but the wheezing has improved. He interprets the CXR as showing some consolidation in the right lower lobe. The parents are experienced in giving the salbutamol and he concludes that Caroline is well enough to go home with a course of oral amoxicillin. The parents are advised to consult their GP if she is no better in a few days time.

Was this a reasonable plan?

Four months later Caroline is referred by the GP to outpatients because of recurrent episodes of high fever,

Avoiding Errors in Paediatrics, First Edition. Joseph E. Raine, Kate Williams and Jonathan Bonser.
© 2013 John Wiley & Sons, Ltd. Published 2013 by Blackwell Publishing Ltd.

cough and anorexia with intermittent wheeze. The GP started her on regular inhaled steroids 2 months earlier, but with no improvement. Her inhaler technique has been assessed as good by the asthma nurse in the surgery. On occasions there has been reduced air entry and crackles at the right base and he mentions the changes reported on the CXR he had requested. Caroline has been given several courses of oral antibiotics which do seem to have helped. On examination she is pale but playing quite happily. Her weight has fallen to between the 2nd and 9th centiles but her height is still following the 25th centile. There is dullness to percussion at the right base with reduced air entry and crackles. A CXR shows collapse and consolidation of the right lower lobe (Case Figure 17.1).

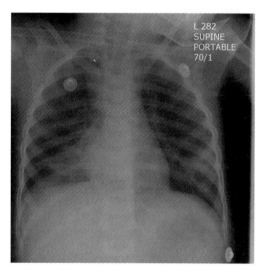

Case Figure 17.1 Caroline's X-ray

The ED CXR is also reported to show these abnormalities and raises the possibility of foreign body inhalation as the changes were also present on the GP's CXR. The consultant also suspects an inhaled foreign body and the nursery staff, when asked, report that she was coughing and spluttering when they found her and acknowledge that she was unsupervised at the time. Caroline is referred for an urgent bronchoscopy and a radiolucent doll's shoe is recovered. She has a prolonged hospital admission for iv antibiotics, physiotherapy and nutrition and has evidence of chronic bronchiectasis and lung fibrosis on a chest CT scan. Caroline's parents write a letter of complaint to the nursery about her lack of supervision and to the hospital about their failure to consider an inhaled foreign body as part of the differ-

ential diagnosis during her ED presentations which has resulted in irreversible lung damage.

Expert opinion

Everything that wheezes isn't asthma or infection induced. Doctors need to stay inquisitive if they are not to fall into the trap of assuming all children have only minor common complaints until proven otherwise. Wheeze is such a common presentation in childhood that rarer causes are easily overlooked in the 'busyness' of an ED and it is tempting to distort the interpretation of symptoms and signs to fit in with a preconceived diagnosis or to limit the differential. As is so frequently the case, the diagnosis revolves around the history which, if inadequate, will miss important clues. Caroline had a sudden onset of cough and wheeze without any symptoms of a viral illness and this should have triggered further questions to the nursery staff specifically exploring the possibility of inhalation. She also had asymmetrical and focal signs. The history from the GP of recurrent chest infections and an abnormal CXR was the second missed opportunity to reach the correct diagnosis. Important information from primary care is all too easily overlooked, especially when children are reviewed by several doctors. The third was the failure of a relatively inexperienced trainee to interpret the second CXR correctly and to compare it with the GP film which would have been available and reported in the computerized storage system. This at the very least should have alerted the team that this problem was chronic and needed more careful thought and discussion with a consultant paediatrician and radiologist. Every department needs a system whereby paediatric staff can discuss films with a radiologist and the latter can draw attention to X-rays that might otherwise escape notice, especially with a rapid turnover of staff and shift patterns of work. A joint X-ray meeting is invaluable. By the time the diagnosis was made Caroline had irreversible lung damage. Even in the absence of a clear history, inhalation of a foreign body should be in the differential diagnosis of recurrent pneumonia.

Legal comment

The hospital staff saw Caroline on three occasions. It may be that an expert can support the treatment and diagnosis reached at the first visit as reasonable. He may comment that a CXR should have been performed, but that the CXR may not have suggested a foreign body.

It will be more difficult to defend the treatment provided on the second visit. This is the key consultation. The expert may conclude that the treatment was suboptimal and that better care would have led to an earlier diagnosis. A respiratory expert would then have to comment on whether removal of the doll's shoe at that time would have saved Caroline from the lung damage that she has suffered.

But the lawyer for the hospital should also investigate the role of the GP. Was the first referral letter appropriate? Did it give sufficient information? Should he have re-referred Caroline earlier? If the GP's actions were not reasonable and his failings caused some of the damage suffered by the girl, then he (through his MDO) would have to contribute to any damages paid.

Further reading and references

Cohen S *et al.* (2009) Suspected foreign body inhalation in children: What are the indications for bronchoscopy?, *The Journal of Paediatrics* 155: 276–80.

 Key learning points

Specific to the case
1. Inhalation of a foreign body should be a differential diagnosis in any child with acute respiratory difficulties, recurrent chest infections and/or persistent CXR changes.
2. Many types of plastic are radiolucent and will not show up on a CXR.

General points
1. Taking a thorough history and staying inquisitive are cornerstones of good clinical practice.
2. A system for reviewing X-rays with a radiologist will help 'mop up' cases that slip through a busy ED with rotating staff and shift patterns of work

Case 18 A jaundiced neonate

Caleb, an 8-day-old infant, is referred by the midwife to the hospital's ED. He is feeding poorly, has lost 800 g, and appears jaundiced.

He was born at full term weighing 3.85 kg by normal vaginal delivery. The pregnancy had been uncomplicated, and he was in good condition at birth. His mother is of black West African ethnicity. Her blood group is O Rhesus Positive.

Caleb was discharged home 12 hours after birth, and was breast fed. His mother had thought he looked jaundiced at 2 days of age, but he appeared to be feeding hungrily and she had not been worried about him at that stage.

On examination, Caleb weighs 3.05 kg and is floppy and lethargic with a dry mouth. His nappy is dry. His capillary refill time is 3 secs, and his feet feel cold. He is apyrexial.

Caleb's abdomen is soft, with a 1 cm liver edge and no other abdominal masses or tenderness. His sclerae, palms and soles appear jaundiced.

What would you do next?

An iv line is sited, and blood is taken for FBC, blood culture, U and Es, blood glucose and bilirubin. Caleb is given a bolus of 20 ml/kg 0.9% sodium chloride.

Initial results phoned to the ED

	Normal
Hb 11 g/dL	13–21 g/dL
WBC 12.5 × 10⁹ /L	5-21 × 10⁹/L
Platelets 320 × 10⁹ /L	150–400 × 10⁹
Total Bilirubin 700 μmol/L	<100 μmol/L
Glucose 3.5 mmol/L	2.8–4.5 mmol/L
Na 146 mmol/L	135–145 mmol/L
K 4.6 mmol/L	3.5–5.0 mmol/L
Urea 9.3 mmol/L	1.1–4.3 mmol/L

A diagnosis of severe neonatal jaundice is made, with sepsis or haemolysis as possible causes. The baby is given iv cefotaxime and amoxicillin.

The local hospital does not have paediatric inpatient beds, and the secondary hospital (5 kilometres away) which normally provides inpatient cover has no paediatric beds. Caleb is therefore transferred to the tertiary hospital, 20 kilometres away, by ambulance, and arrives there 5 hours following his initial presentation to the local hospital.

What are your priorities for this baby?

Shortly after arrival at the tertiary hospital, Caleb has a short, self-terminating generalized seizure lasting 2 minutes. Blood glucose, calcium and blood gases are normal.

Caleb is placed under double phototherapy lights, rehydrated with 10% dextrose/0.45% sodium chloride, and blood is urgently cross matched for a double volume exchange blood transfusion.

Peripheral arterial access is obtained.

Laboratory results at the tertiary hospital
- Total bilirubin 840 μmol/L
- Blood group A, Rhesus Positive
- Direct Antiglobulin Test (DAT): Positive

An isovolaemic, double volume (160 ml/kg) exchange blood transfusion is performed. The procedure starts 6 hours after the initial presentation, 20 ml of blood are replaced by the peripheral venous line every 4 minutes whilst the same volume is removed via the peripheral arterial line. Caleb has continuous ECG and temperature monitoring, and BP is recorded after each 80 mls of blood transfused. During the procedure, he has two further brief seizures.

At the end of the procedure:
- Total bilirubin 260 μmol/L
- Hb 16.3 g/dL, WBC 14.4 × 10⁹/L, Platelets 64 × 10⁹/L

Avoiding Errors in Paediatrics, First Edition. Joseph E. Raine, Kate Williams and Jonathan Bonser.
© 2013 John Wiley & Sons, Ltd. Published 2013 by Blackwell Publishing Ltd.

- Total calcium 2.1 mmol/L (2.2–2.7 mmol/L)
- Glucose 4.0 mmol/L

What further investigations are important?

Because of the seizures, a cerebral US is performed, followed by a LP.

Cerebral ultrasound:
- Normal intracranial anatomy. No intracranial bleeding.

Lumbar puncture:
- Xanthochromic CSF
- 2 WBC, 100 RBC
- No bacterial growth after 48hr incubation in blood or CSF.

Caleb continues under phototherapy lights for a further 2 days. He is fed expressed breast milk after 12 hours, by a nasogastric tube. The following day, Glucose 6 Phosphate Dehydrogenase (G6PD) enzyme deficiency is reported. The blood platelet count rises spontaneously to 180×10^9 /L after 48 hours.

Follow-up of hearing at 4 weeks and 3 months of age demonstrates severe sensorineural deafness. Caleb becomes progressively dystonic, and at 18 months of age is microcephalic, with clear clinical evidence of athetoid cerebral palsy.

The final diagnosis is kernicterus secondary to haemolytic jaundice as a result of combined ABO incompatibility and G6PD deficiency.

Caleb's family complain stating that the delay in performing the exchange transfusion has led to their son's cerebral palsy, and that they had not been warned of the dangers of jaundice in the newborn.

 Expert opinion

The diagnosis of jaundice can be a difficult clinical task in infants with pigmented skin. It is therefore important to have a low clinical threshold for obtaining a blood bilirubin measurement if there is any clinical suspicion of jaundice. The trend of early hospital discharges for babies who appear well at birth has resulted in jaundiced babies presenting in the community. Midwives should inform mothers about jaundice which is very common in newborns (although kernicterus is very rare). Jaundice is one of the commonest reasons for readmission to hospital of babies in the first week of life.

Severe jaundice is usually a result of a haemolytic process or of neonatal sepsis. In this case there was ABO blood group incompatibility, with evidence of IgG coating of the infant's red blood cells (DAT positivity). A second cause of haemolysis was the presence of G6PD deficiency, which renders red blood cells more susceptible to oxidative injury. G6PD deficiency is inherited in a sex-linked manner (carried by the mother, with a 50% likelihood of expression in a male child) and is commoner in people of Mediterranean and black African ancestry – a jaundiced male black African infant has approximately a 35% chance of having G6PD deficiency.

Severe neonatal jaundice is a medical emergency. Blood taken at the local hospital should have been sent by courier to the regional blood transfusion centre for cross match to expedite treatment. If phototherapy units were available in the local hospital than this treatment should have been started immediately whilst awaiting an exchange transfusion, which should have been initiated in an expeditious fashion. The presenting bilirubin measurement at the local hospital was well above the exchange transfusion threshold of 450 μmol/L recommended in the NICE Guidance for babies over 42 hours old, and there was a prolonged delay in initiating effective treatment of the jaundice. In this case, the first seizure on arrival at the tertiary hospital, was thought to be due to symptomatic bilirubin encephalopathy.

 Legal comment

There seem to have been a number of breaches of duty in this case, by various parts of the NHS, leading to a disastrous delay.

- The antenatal service and/or hospital nurses may not have adequately informed the mother on her discharge of some common neonatal conditions such as jaundice.
- The midwife who would have visited the home every 1-2 days seems not to have taken adequate note of the baby's jaundice. Early signs seem to have been missed as by the time the midwife did refer the baby to hospital at 8 days, he was obviously very jaundiced.
- That hospital carried out the correct investigations and made the correct diagnosis, but did not instigate emergency treatment. Blood taken at the local hospital was not sent for an urgent cross match. Did the local hospital have facilities for immediate phototherapy? Phototherapy should have been started as soon as possible. Was the tertiary hospital told of the urgency of the situation before the baby arrived?

This sequence of events led to considerable delays and makes it inevitable that this case will be settled. Caleb's cerebral palsy will undoubtedly be shown to be due to the delays and the damages will be very considerable.

 Key learning points

Specific to the case

1. Severe neonatal jaundice is a medical emergency.
2. Babies with pigmented skin can be more difficult to assess.
3. Ethnicity and gender may affect the risk of illness.
4. Parents are the first line of defence for newborn babies. It is important that they are aware of significant risks for their baby in the first few days of life, especially when they are discharged home shortly after the birth.

General points

1. Record counselling discussions in the patient's medical notes.
2. Delays in patient transfer between hospitals may impact on outcomes. Record the reasons for any significant delay, and ensure that you participate fully in audits of transferred cases.

Further reading and references

National Collaborating Centre for Women's and Children's Health, Royal College of Obstetricians and Gynaecologists (2010) Neonatal Jaundice Clinical Guideline.

National Institute for Clinical Excellence (2010) Recognition and Treatment of Neonatal Jaundice. http://www.nice.org.uk/CG98

Case 19 A febrile boy with a limp

Fawad, a 4-year-old boy visiting the UK from Pakistan, presents to the ED at 3pm on a Sunday with a fever and limping. The FY2 doctor in ED takes a history from mum, who speaks little English. This reveals that Fawad had a minor fall in the park 5 days ago and developed a fever of 39°C 3 days ago. He has been complaining of pain in his right leg for 48 hours, and is now refusing to weight bear. The FY2 doctor bleeps the Paediatric ST1 doctor, as she is unable to examine Fawad, who screams whenever she touches him.

What would you do now?

The ST1 takes a limited history also without an interpreter. He tries to examine the child, but Fawad is crying and fighting him off. He attempts to take blood but is unsuccessful and stops as Fawad is becoming very distressed. At 5.45pm the ST1 contacts the Paediatric registrar, who is busy on the neonatal unit, and advises oral analgesia and hip X-rays. The ST1 also calls the orthopaedic ST2, who says he will review the child with the X-ray results.

What is your differential diagnosis?

The Paediatric ST1 is concerned about the possibility of a septic arthritis, but feels that the X-rays are normal and is reassured now that Fawad has settled down following analgesia. Examination of Fawad is normal and there is no deformity, swelling or erythema of the right leg. However, Fawad still cries when the right hip is examined and he refuses to walk. The ST1 doctor now feels that the diagnosis is more likely to be a transient synovitis. He is aware that Fawad has been in the ED for nearly 4 hours and that the mother is keen to go home to her other children. On discussion with his registrar he decides to discharge the child with ibuprofen prior to the orthopaedic review, and to see him on the day unit in 2 days.

Do you agree with this management plan?

Fawad re-presents to the ED on Tuesday morning, accompanied by his mother and an English relative, concerned that he is still febrile and in more pain. They are referred directly to the paediatric registrar who is worried about the right hip. She takes blood for culture, FBC, CRP and ESR, and contacts the orthopaedic registrar, who advises holding off antibiotics until their review. The orthopaedic team see him on the ward with blood results that show a WCC of 18.3×10^9/L (normal $4–12 \times 10^9$/L) with 15.7×10^9/L neutrophils (normal $1.5–6.0 \times 10^9$/L), CRP of 176 mg/L (normal<6 mg/L) and ESR of 92 mm/h (normal <10 mm/h). They arrange a hip ultrasound that afternoon which demonstrates a significant joint effusion. In view of the risk of a septic arthritis they proceed to an arthrotomy under general anaesthetic later that evening and remove significant amounts of infected material from the joint. Microscopy of the joint fluid shows gram positive bacteria, and grows *Staphylococcus aureus* after 24 hours.

Fawad's temperatures settle after 48 hours but he continues to complain of pain and requires analgesia, a prolonged course of intravenous antibiotics and physiotherapy. After discharge a MRI scan reveals changes consistent with avascular necrosis of the hip and he requires further surgery; despite this his limp persists. Fawad's family complain, stating that if the infection had been diagnosed at the first presentation his subsequent problems would have been avoided.

Expert opinion

The presentation of fever with a limp in a child (3–10 years) is very common and is usually due to transient synovitis. However, septic arthritis must be considered, particularly in children with high fevers and refusal to weight bear. Joint infections are notoriously difficult to diagnose and plain radiographs are usually normal,

---

Avoiding Errors in Paediatrics, First Edition. Joseph E. Raine, Kate Williams and Jonathan Bonser.
© 2013 John Wiley & Sons, Ltd. Published 2013 by Blackwell Publishing Ltd.

but necessary to exclude traumatic injury, a diagnosis of Perthe's disease or a slipped upper femoral epiphysis in an older child. Kocher's algorithm includes 4 criteria to distinguish septic arthritis from transient synovitis: refusal to weight-bear; fever $>38.5°C$; ESR >40 mm/h; and WCC $>12.0 \times 10^9$/L. The probability of a joint infection rises from $<0.2\%$ with none of these features, to 99% if all four are present. In this case the failure of the paediatric ST1 to do blood tests, compounded by the lack of senior paediatric or orthopaedic review at presentation and the delay in review until 2 days later, led to a delay in diagnosis and treatment. Late treatment, five or more days after onset of symptoms, is associated with a high incidence of sequelae such as avascular necrosis or damage to the growth plate, whereas cases treated promptly have an excellent outcome.

 Legal comment

This case will prove indefensible and should be settled as soon as possible. There was a clear failure to diagnose the problem and earlier intervention would probably have prevented the damage to the hip.

The language barrier meant that it was difficult for the ST1 to obtain a good history. But attempts should have been made to find an interpreter. A judge is unlikely to excuse this failing.

Further reading and references

Howard A, Wilson M (2010) Easily missed? Septic arthritis in children. *BMJ* 341: c4407.

Kocher MS, Mandiga R, Zurakowski D, Barnewolt C, Kasser JR (2004) Validation of a clinical prediction rule for the differentiation between septic arthritis and transient synovitis of the hip in children. *J Bone Joint Surg (Am)* 86: 1629–35.

Nunn TR, Cheung WY, Rollinson PD (2007) A prospective study of pyogenic sepsis of the hip in childhood. *J Bone Joint Surg (Br)* 89: 100–6.

Schwentker E (2009) Septic arthritis; Paediatrics. http://emedicine.medscape.com/article/1259337-overview

 Key learning points

Specific to the case

1. Transient synovitis is the commonest cause of childhood limp. However, other possibilities such as septic arthritis and osteomyelitis must be considered, particularly in children with high fevers and refusal to weight bear, as prompt diagnosis is vital to prevent permanent problems.

2. Septic arthritis presents in the hip in a third of paediatric cases and most commonly affects children less than 5 years of age.

3. Blood tests are necessary in the investigation of possible septic arthritis as they are very useful in diagnosis in conjunction with clinical features (Kocher's red flags).

4. Preschool children are often difficult to examine thoroughly. This child seemed 'difficult' because he was in pain, which was a significant sign in itself. Re-examination following analgesia can be very helpful. Where problems persist a senior review should be requested.

General points

1. Language barriers have a significant impact on the ability of doctors to take a history. Whenever possible interpreter services should be used and doctors need to be aware that they may be held responsible for diagnostic failures due to incomplete history taking.

2. Reviewing the patient is an important diagnostic tool; where the diagnosis is unclear, admission to the ward or a repeat appointment within 24 hours may be required.

3. Paediatric referrals, especially out-of-hours, are best made to the Paediatric registrar so that urgent cases can be prioritized; the hospital should consider instituting this policy.

4. Innovations such as the 4 hour time limit in ED have been very helpful but should never prevent a patient getting the appropriate treatment.

5. The hospital should consider having a separate general and neonatal registrar rota.

Case 20 A febrile neonate

Kai, a 3-week-old infant, presents to the emergency department at 9.30 am on a Sunday morning with a 1 day history of feeling hot, poor feeding, and occasional jerky movements. He has a temperature of 38.3°C, is quite lethargic and is observed to have some jerky movements of his left arm which last for a few seconds only. The nurse bleeps the paediatric ST1 doctor who has only done 5 weeks of paediatrics.

What would you do now?

The ST1 states that she is busy on the ward round and asks the nurse to get the ED's FY2 doctor to see the patient first. The patient is seen by the FY2 who is concerned about the possibility of serious sepsis and he contacts the paediatric ST1 asking her to review the baby. The ST1 states that she has nearly finished the ward round and will come soon. Kai is seen by the paediatric ST1 at 12.30 pm. She observes that he has a brief 5-second apnoea. Kai has no rash, has a flat anterior fontanelle and no neck stiffness.

What is your differential diagnosis?

The ST1's diagnosis is a septic neonate who requires a septic screen. Her differential diagnosis lists septicaemia, meningitis, pneumonia and a urinary tract infection.

Kai is transferred to the paediatric ward for a septic screen but the ST1 doctor is unable to get any blood and calls the registrar. The registrar who has so far been unaware of this baby and who is covering general paediatrics and neonates arrives at 3 pm. A urine dipstick has been done and is negative for nitrites with only a trace of leucocytes. A CXR is normal. He is concerned about the possibility of meningitis and that the jerky arm movements and the apnoeas have in fact been fits. He obtains a FBC, CRP, U and E's, bone chemistry, LFTs, a blood culture and a glucose. The glucose is 1.9 mmol/L (normal 2.8–4.5 mmol/L) and he administers a 2 ml/kg, 10% dextrose bolus injection following which the glu-

cose level normalizes. He performs a LP which reveals cloudy CSF and calls his consultant who recommends intravenous penicillin and gentamicin. The antibiotics are administered at 5 pm.

The LP shows a WBC of 1867/mm^3 (normal ≤ 20/mm^3) of which 90% are polymorphs, a protein of 3.2 g/L (normal < 0.7 g/L) and a glucose of 0.9 mmol/L (normal >60% simultaneous blood glucose). On microscopy Gram positive cocci are seen consistent with a diagnosis of Group B streptococcal meningitis.

At 6 pm Kai has a seizure with cyanosis, loss of consciousness and rhythmic arm movements lasting 7 minutes.

What treatment would you give?

An intravenous loading dose of phenobarbitone is administered and maintenance phenobarbitone is prescribed. Over the next few days the fits continue. An EEG is markedly abnormal and a MRI scan shows areas of infection, infarction and cerebral oedema.

Kai subsequently develops cerebral palsy with a hemiplegia, learning difficulties, deafness and epilepsy.

Kai's parents complain and subsequently sue. They state that there was an unacceptable delay in the administration of antibiotics and that prompt treatment would have prevented or significantly diminished the neurological sequelae.

Do you think the parents will succeed in their claim?

 ## Expert opinion

A fever ≥ 38°C in a neonate is a medical emergency. The ST1 doctor should have appreciated the urgency of the problem and prioritized her work appropriately. Sepsis in neonates can present in nonspecific ways such as fever, poor feeding and lethargy. Fits in neonates can present in subtle ways and the abnormal jerky arm movements and apnoeas should certainly have prompted the ST1

Avoiding Errors in Paediatrics, First Edition. Joseph E. Raine, Kate Williams and Jonathan Bonser.
© 2013 John Wiley & Sons, Ltd. Published 2013 by Blackwell Publishing Ltd.

doctor to consider that the infant may be fitting. A bulging anterior fontanelle is a late sign in neonatal meningitis. Neck stiffness is an extremely poor sign in neonates as they in any case have poor head control and are often floppy when ill. Furthermore, the ST1 doctor should have discussed this case with her registrar following the phone call from the ED nurse. If the registrar was unable to come immediately after being contacted about this case due to other urgent work he should have phoned his consultant to obtain the necessary help. The delay of 7.5 hours between the child presenting to the ED and receiving antibiotics is unacceptably long. It is highly likely that Kai would have had neurological sequelae even with prompt treatment but the delay in the administration of antibiotics is likely to have been partially responsible for the subsequent morbidity.

 Legal comment

The care provided to Kai was substandard and treatment should have been commenced earlier. A full valuation of the case could run to two or three million pounds, if it could be shown that all Kai's injuries were caused by the delay. But the Expert Opinion indicates that this child would probably have suffered some neurological sequelae, even if he had been treated earlier. Kai's family will have to show to what extent he has been affected by the negligence. If there would have been no practical difference in the outcome, then the claim will fail.

If, however, earlier treatment would have made a material difference, then compensation will be calculated to take account of the poorer outcome. The final figure could be anywhere between low tens of thousands to more than a million pounds, depending on the nature of the reports obtained by the hospital and the family.

Further reading and references

Dredge DC, Krishnamoorthy KS (2010) Neonatal Meningitis. http://emedicine.medscape.com/article/1176960-overview

Meningitis Research Foundation (2011) Useful source of information on meningitis and septicaemia for health professionals and the public. http://www.meningitis.org

National Institute of Clinical Excellence (2007) Feverish Illness in Children – Assessment and Initial Management in Children Younger than 5 Years. http://www.nice.org.uk/cg047

 Key learning points

Specific to the case
1. A fever of 38°C or more in a neonate should be dealt with urgently.
2. It is always important to consider meningitis in the differential diagnosis of a febrile neonate as it is a very serious but treatable disease.
3. Neonatal sepsis can present with very nonspecific signs, for example poor feeding.
4. Fits can present in subtle, atypical ways, for example apnoeas.
5. Severe sepsis can lead to hypoglycaemia and a blood glucose should always be performed in fitting children.
6. Neck stiffness is a useful sign in older children but is a poor sign in infants <1 year of age.
7. A febrile neonate should have a full septic screen prior to starting intravenous antibiotics. If the infant is not well enough to undergo a LP than the antibiotics should be commenced and the LP can be done when the child is better. Occasionally, if the child is not tachypnoeic and there are no respiratory signs then the CXR can be omitted. If required, the CXR can be done after the antibiotics have been started. If a urine sample cannot be obtained than a suprapubic aspirate should be attempted. If that fails, than urine should be collected after starting antibiotics and the there should be a low threshold for performing a renal US if a urinary tract infection is subsequently suspected to be the cause of the sepsis. The septic screen should be done promptly and the antibiotics should be administered as soon as possible.

General points
1. The National Institute for Clinical Excellence (NICE) has published a 1 page 'traffic light' system to help assess the likelihood of serious disease in febrile children. It is recommended that this is displayed in all emergency departments and paediatric wards.
2. It is important for junior doctors to prioritise their work correctly and to know their limitations.
3. The hospital should review its referral guidelines. A guideline stating that all referrals from the ED and admissions to the ward must be discussed with the registrar (or if they are unavailable the consultant on call) would help avoid delays in diagnosis and treatment.

Case 21 A neonate with abnormal movements

A 3-week-old boy, Oliver, presents to the ED on Friday morning with abnormal movements. His mother noticed abnormal movements of the arms on one occasion and of one leg on another. Oliver seems unresponsive when having these episodes. There is no cyanosis and the longest episode has lasted for 30 seconds. There have been 6 episodes in the past 24 hours. Oliver has not had a fever but has been feeding less well than usual and has also been lethargic.

His mother was well in pregnancy and he was born by vaginal delivery following an uneventful labour. There was no prolonged rupture of membranes.

Oliver's mother is not on medication and there is no history of drug abuse. The parents are not consanguineous.

On examination Oliver has a temperature of 37.9°C, a saturation of 97% in air and is not dehydrated. There is no rash. The anterior fontanelle is flat and there are no neurological signs. There are no signs in the other systems.

A bedside blood glucose is 4.3 mmol/L. The registrar who sees an episode feels that Oliver is fitting and discusses him with the consultant.

What investigations and treatment would you recommend?

The consultant suggests doing a full septic screen excluding a CXR (Oliver has no respiratory symptoms or signs), U and E's, bone chemistry, Mg, LFTs, a laboratory glucose and to subsequently start iv penicillin and gentamicin.

The lumbar puncture is performed but only 3 drops of CSF are obtained. The CSF result is as follows:

- WBC 290/mm³ (normal ≤ 20/mm³) of which 70% are polymorphs
- RBC 18/mm³
- Gram stain – negative

- Rapid antigen screen – negative
- Protein 1.8 g/L (normal < 0.7 g/L)
- Glucose 2.0 mmol/L (normal >60% simultaneous blood glucose).

The microbiology technician who phones the ward with the result states that because the sample was so small the figures are approximate and the Gram stain can sometimes be negative in cases of bacterial meningitis, especially with small samples.

What is your opinion of the CSF result?

Oliver continues to fit and is given a loading dose of phenobarbitone. The following morning he is still having intermittent fits.

What further treatment would you give for the fits?

Oliver is given a loading dose of phenytoin and commenced on regular iv phenobarbitone. Intravenous lorazepam is used for the episodic fits that occur during the day. A CT scan is performed and is normal. On Sunday evening, over 48 hours following admission, Oliver develops status epilepticus and requires intubation, ventilation and transfer to a PICU. There he is also given iv aciclovir. On Monday morning the CSF PCR returns as positive for type 2 herpes and a diagnosis of herpes encephalitis is made. Oliver's parents are specifically asked about a history of herpes genitalis. Both state that they have not had this but they are referred to a genitourinary clinic where serological tests confirm that they both have antibodies to herpes type 2 and therefore must have had this infection in the past. Oliver returns to the local hospital, having been successfully extubated but 10 days later again develops status epilepticus and requires re-intubation, ventilation and another transfer to the PICU.

Avoiding Errors in Paediatrics, First Edition. Joseph E. Raine, Kate Williams and Jonathan Bonser.
© 2013 John Wiley & Sons, Ltd. Published 2013 by Blackwell Publishing Ltd.

EEG shows marked epileptiform activity and a MRI shows widespread cystic leucomalacia. Oliver subsequently develops severe learning difficulties.

His parents sue because of the delay in the diagnosis of the herpes encephalitis and the resultant complications.

 Expert opinion

Herpes encephalitis is rare. In cases due to vertical transmission it usually occurs between 4 and 11 days of age, but can present as late as 4 weeks. Oliver's mother should have been discreetly, specifically asked about a history of genital herpes but in most infants who present with this condition there is no clinical history of this illness even though the mother has serological evidence of the disease. In approximately 40% of cases there are no herpetic skin lesions.

In an older child a focal fit would have the same significance as a focal neurological sign and would make one consider a condition such as herpes encephalitis or a structural brain lesion. However, fits in neonates can be quite subtle and may appear to be focal even in cases where there is a more generalized problem such as meningitis. In some cases of bacterial meningitis, especially if there is little CSF to analyse, the Gram stain can be negative and the diagnosis may be made subsequently on the more sensitive culture or PCR. Though sometimes one does not see organisms on a Gram stain this is unusual and should have prompted the doctors to think of nonbacterial causes of meningitis or encephalitis. Though the CSF white blood cell differential suggests a bacterial cause, early on in viral meningitis there can be a predominance of polymorphs and in this case the result was in any case approximate due to the small sample size. The CSF glucose is often normal in viral meningitis but can be low as in this case. Furthermore, the rapid antigen screen was negative. The administration of aciclovir should therefore have been considered following the CSF result.

Oliver's worsening condition should also have made the doctors review the diagnosis prior to the onset of status epilepticus on Sunday. However, whether this would have made a difference to the long-term outcome is difficult to determine.

Aciclovir is a very safe drug and where there is doubt about the diagnosis it is safer to administer it and to then discontinue it if the patient improves and the CSF herpes PCR proves to be negative. It would have been wise to discuss this rare case with a consultant microbiologist and/or a tertiary infectious diseases centre.

 Legal comment

The Expert Opinion above shows that this is a complex, difficult case. The clinicians did start treatment quickly. They seem to have acted reasonably. However, an instructed expert may criticize them for failing to consider herpes encephalitis as a differential diagnosis. The real issue is whether aciclovir should have been administered earlier and whether, on the balance of probabilities, it would have prevented the child from developing learning difficulties. If the answer is 'yes' to both these questions, then the case could be worth several million pounds.

Whether the clinicians were negligent or not, a mistake was made. The case should, therefore, be viewed as an important lesson in considering all potential diagnoses.

 Key learning points

Specific to the case
1. In most infants with a diagnosis of herpes encephalitis there is no history of maternal herpes.
2. In the absence of organisms on Gram stain in the CSF it is safer to administer iv aciclovir until the CSF viral PCR is known.
3. In viral meningitis there can initially be a predominance of polymorphs.
4. It is advisable to discuss rare and complex infectious diseases with a consultant in microbiology or infectious diseases.

General points
1. One should not shy away from asking questions about sensitive issues such as genitourinary infections.
2. If a patient fails to improve as anticipated than the diagnosis should be reviewed.

Further reading and references

Pinninti SG, Tolan RW (2010) 2. Herpes Simplex Virus Infection. http://emedicine.medscape.com/article/964866-overview

Sheth RD (2009) Neonatal Seizures. http://emedicine.medscape.com/article/1177069-overview

Tidy C (2010) Herpes Simplex Encephalitis. http://www.patient.co.uk/doctor/Herpes-Encephalitis.htm

Case 22 A teenager with scrotal pain

Adam, a 15-year-old boy, presents to the ED at 10 pm with a 4-hour history of severe right-sided testicular pain. There is no history of any injury or of recent infections. He has no genitourinary symptoms, has never had a urinary tract infection and is not sexually active. He is apyrexial and has an erythematous, swollen scrotum with marked tenderness and swelling of the testes (Case Figure 22.1). The FY2 in the ED department is concerned about the possibility of testicular torsion and calls the surgical ST2 who is also covering urology. The surgical ST2 is busy with a sick patient in the intensive care unit. He tells the FY2 that the urology registrar is on call from home and not in the hospital and asks the FY2 to contact the paediatric team.

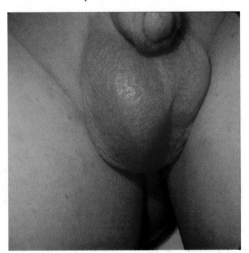

Case Figure 22.1 The appearance of Adam's scrotum. Reproduced with permission from Hutson et al. (2007). *Jones' Clinical Paediatric Surgery*, thedn. Wiley-Blackwell, Oxford.

Do you agree with the surgical ST2's approach?

The paediatric ST3 sees Adam, who is clearly in pain. The urine dipstick shows leucocytes++. The paediatric

doctor is also concerned about the possibility of torsion and calls the surgical ST2. The ST2 is still busy, states that the patient may have epididymitis or orchitis and asks the paediatric ST3 to admit Adam to the paediatric ward, prescribe analgesia and arrange an urgent scrotal US for the following morning.

What would you have done?

At 8.30 the following morning Adam is seen by the urology registrar who makes a clinical diagnosis of testicular torsion, cancels the US and arranges urgent surgery to explore the scrotum. In theatre, the left testis is found to be necrotic and is removed and a right sided orchidoplexy is performed.

Adam's mother complains and later sues the hospital because of the delay in the diagnosis, stating that the testis could have been saved if the diagnosis and treatment had been quicker.

Expert opinion

The diagnosis of testicular torsion is primarily a clinical one and in two-thirds of cases the diagnosis can be made from the history and examination alone. There is no need for a scrotal US if clinically the diagnosis is clear. In fact, ordering an US under these circumstances may lead to unnecessary and deleterious delay. If the operation is carried out in less than 6 hours from the onset of symptoms there is a 90–100% chance of saving the testis, beyond 12 hours the chances are 20–50%. Over 24 hours the chance of salvaging the testis is close to 0%. A scrotal US should only be done in doubtful cases.

Epididymitis and epididymo-orchitis are differential diagnosis of testicular torsion. These conditions most commonly occur as a result of reflux of infected urine into the epididymis, or from the sexually acquired diseases caused by chlamydia or gonococcus. The history in these cases is of a more gradual onset of pain, often

---

Avoiding Errors in Paediatrics, First Edition. Joseph E. Raine, Kate Williams and Jonathan Bonser.
© 2013 John Wiley & Sons, Ltd. Published 2013 by Blackwell Publishing Ltd.

developing over several days, rather than a few hours of the sudden, severe pain that typifies torsion. Epididymitis and epididymo-orchitis are often accompanied by systemic symptoms such as a fever, symptoms of a urinary tract infection and in some cases a urethral discharge. There may be leucocytes in the urine (25%) and a bacterial growth. However, in 30% of cases of torsion the urine analysis will also show leucocytes, so that this finding may not help differentiate between the above conditions. Orchitis is a further differential of torsion that is most commonly a complication of mumps.

The history and examination in this case are typical of testicular torsion, a common emergency that the surgical ST2 should have known more about. He was also wrong to ignore the concerns of the ED FY2 and the paediatric ST3 who had actually seen the patient. This case comprises a clear urological emergency and in this setting the surgical ST2, as he was very busy, should have obtained the help of the urology registrar or consultant. It was inappropriate and a waste of valuable time to involve the paediatric team. The nature and extent of his supervision should also be looked into. Fortunately, one testis is sufficient to maintain fertility.

 Legal comment

This case needs to be settled as soon as possible. The hospital has clearly failed to treat Adam appropriately and an expert is likely to conclude that earlier treatment would have saved the testicle. The damages will be in the region of £15,000.

A lawyer would tend to look at the mistakes of individual doctors, but this case clearly reveals failings in the systems in place at the hospital. The Key Learning Points below comment on the lack of guidelines for when junior doctors should discuss cases with their seniors and questions the supervision arrangements. But it also mentions something else: respect for the views of other doctors. If the surgical ST2 had listened to the concerns of the paediatric ST3 and FY2, Adam would probably have not lost his testicle. Arrogance and failure to listen to the concerns of others are issues that may need addressing with the surgical ST2 to prevent further errors.

 Key learning points

Specific to the case

1. Unilateral testicular pain is due to testicular torsion until proven otherwise. The diagnosis is usually a clinical one. A scrotal US should only be done in doubtful cases. Due to the risk of testicular infarction and necrosis, treatment is urgent.

2. In torsion pain is sudden and severe and the history is typically one of a few hours. In contrast, in epididymitis and epididymo-orchitis the pain is more gradual, often developing over several days, there is frequently a fever and genitourinary symptoms.

General points

1. Junior doctors should be familiar with the initial management of emergencies in their speciality.

2. In the case of a clear urological emergency, such as a possible testicular torsion, if the junior doctor is too busy to see the patient promptly they should seek the help of a more senior doctor in the same speciality. There should be clear departmental guidelines as to which cases should be discussed with a registrar and/or consultant in all specialities.

3. A doctor should have greater respect and pay more attention to the repeated concerns of medical colleagues, even if they work in a different speciality.

4. Procedures regarding supervision should be reviewed. For instance, it would be wise for a registrar and/or consultant to phone the junior doctor in the hospital between 11pm and 12 midnight to discuss any urgent or complex patients.

Further reading and references

Minevich E, McQuiston LT (2010) Testicular torsion. http://emedicine.medscape.com/article/438817-overview

Sabanegh ED, Ching CB (2010) Epididymitis. http://emedicine.medscape.com/article/436154-overview

Case 23 A boy with nonspecific symptoms

Asil, a 7-year-old Turkish boy, has a fever and a runny nose. He becomes 'lifeless and lethargic' and is taken to the GP. His parents speak limited English so it is difficult to get a clear history. Blood tests are requested and show a normal Hb, WCC and platelet count. The CRP is 20 (normal <6 mg/L), there are atypical mononuclear cells on the blood film and the monospot is positive.

What is the likely diagnosis?

The GP makes a diagnosis of glandular fever.

A week later Asil is brought back to the GP. He has developed bad headaches which keep him awake at night despite paracetamol and ibuprofen. He is vomiting and this is getting worse. He does not have diarrhoea. The GP feels that the symptoms are compatible with glandular fever, prescribes dioralyte and reassures the family.

What should be done now?

About 3 weeks later Asil's parents bring him to the ED one evening. Again there is a language barrier which makes obtaining the history difficult. Asil's headaches are worse and he is still vomiting frequently. Examination by a FY2 ED doctor does not reveal any abnormalities but it is noted that Asil has lost weight, 2 kg in approximately 3 weeks. His symptoms are again thought to be due to glandular fever and he is sent home and the family are advised to continue with the analgesia and to keep Asil well hydrated.

What are your concerns at this point?

Two weeks later the GP refers Asil to the paediatric rapid referral clinic where he is seen by the consultant paediatrician. He still has headaches and vomiting. On examination Asil is miserable and thin. He is thought to be slightly dehydrated and has a central capillary refill time of 3–4 seconds. There is no fever, no lymphadenopathy and no rash. No abnormalities are detected in the respiratory or cardiovascular systems. His abdomen is scaphoid, soft and nontender. There is no organomegaly. He has no neck stiffness.

What is the differential diagnosis now?

Asil is admitted to the day unit for a fluid challenge. The plan is that if the fluid challenge fails he will require iv fluids and that blood tests will be done when the cannula is inserted. Asil has a urine dipstick which is normal and 2 hourly observations. Whilst on the day unit he vomits several times and complains of a severe headache. There is a family history of migraine.

He is examined by the paediatric ST1 who cannot see the fundi, documents that the cranial nerves are normal, finds power, tone, and coordination to be normal but thinks that the knee and ankle jerks are too brisk and that there is bilateral ankle clonus.

Asil is then examined by a registrar who confirms the pathologically brisk reflexes and the clonus in the ankles.

What should happen next?

Asil has an urgent CT brain scan (Case Figure 23.1)

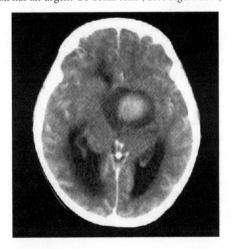

Case Figure 23.1 Asil's CT scan

Avoiding Errors in Paediatrics, First Edition. Joseph E. Raine, Kate Williams and Jonathan Bonser.
© 2013 John Wiley & Sons, Ltd. Published 2013 by Blackwell Publishing Ltd.

The postcontrast CT shows a mass lying to the left of the midline at the level of the 3rd ventricle, showing central enhancement and surrounding oedema with associated obstructive dilatation of the lateral ventricles.

Asil is referred to the tertiary oncology and neurosurgical centre. A biopsy shows a low grade astrocytic tumour. He requires an external ventricular drain as an emergency procedure. A subsequent MRI scan shows involvement of the left optic nerve. The shunt is later internalized. Complete surgical resection is not possible. Radiotherapy is considered the best option in terms of stopping tumour growth but is not given due to the serious potential side effects. Instead Asil is treated with chemotherapy for 18 months. At follow-up he is found to have very poor vision in his left eye, behaviour problems and is struggling at school.

His parents complain, stating that the diagnosis should have been made sooner and that doing so would have alleviated some of the resultant morbidity.

 Expert opinion

Asil's illness began with nonspecific symptoms which could have been due to a multitude of mild childhood viral infections. The parents' limited English may have made it more difficult to get a clear history, so it was even more important that the child be thoroughly examined and re-evaluated when he was getting worse rather than recovering from his viral infection. The initial investigations requested by the GP and the initial diagnosis were reasonable, but in retrospect too much reliance was placed on the positive monospot result (which in any case has a poor sensitivity and specificity) instead of re-evaluating Asil in the light of his new symptoms of a severe headache and vomiting which are not common in glandular fever. These new symptoms should have prompted a thorough neurological examination, consideration of the possibility of a cranial space occupying lesion and referral to the hospital. An earlier neurological examination would probably have elicited the upper motor neurone signs in the legs (brisk reflexes and clonus) which were highly suggestive of a space occupying lesion in the brain. The use of a translating service at the GP's or in the ED would have facilitated the history taking and may have sped up the diagnosis.

 Legal comment

An investigation of the parents' complaint is likely to highlight the possibility of error by both their GP and the hospital's ED. The parents may then see a solicitor about the prospects of litigation. That solicitor will have to take expert opinions on a number of questions. Firstly, whether it was negligent of their GP and the FY2 doctor in the ED not to have done a neurological examination sooner than they did? Secondly, if they had done such an examination, what would they probably have found? Thirdly, if appropriate management had been initiated at that point, what would the outcome have been for Asil? The Expert Opinion above says that '*in retrospect* too much reliance was placed on the positive monospot result'. It is an abiding problem for experts to try to eliminate hindsight from their judgement of a case scenario, and to put themselves in the position of the clinician at the time.

We are told that Asil now has poor vision in his left eye and behavioural problems. Although the standard of care may be criticized by their expert, the family may well still have problems proving that earlier treatment would have improved the outcome.

 Key learning points

Specific to the case
• The early signs of cancer can be subtle and initially indistinguishable from common childhood illnesses. However, severe headaches with vomiting should always raise alarm bells and prompt a full neurological examination.
• The assumption was made by a number of doctors that glandular fever was the cause of his symptoms. There was an over reliance on test results and a failure to keep an open mind about the diagnosis. Severe headaches and vomiting are not common symptoms in glandular fever.
• Failure to recognize 'red flag' symptoms:
  ○ headache keeping a patient awake at night
  ○ headache not responding to paracetamol or ibuprofen
  ○ significant weight loss.
• A translating service should be used when there is a language barrier

General points
• The NICE guidelines state that an urgent referral to hospital should be made when a child or young person is seen by the GP (or in ED) three times with the same problem with no clear diagnosis being made.

- It can be very difficult to do a neurological examination on a young child who is in pain or unwell. In such cases there should be a lower threshold for requesting a brain scan (CT or ideally MRI).

Further reading and references

HeadSmart (2011) Be Brain Tumour Aware. www. headsmart.org.uk

NICE (2005) Referral guidelines for suspected cancer. http://www.nice.org.uk/nicemedia/pdf/CG27publicinfo

Wilne S, Koller K, Collier J *et al*. The diagnosis of brain tumours in children: a guideline to assist healthcare professionals in the assessment of children who may have a brain tumour. *Arch Dis Child* 95: 534–9. http://adc.bmj.com/content/95/7/534.abstract

Case 24 A delayed walker

A female infant, Natalie, is born by normal vaginal delivery at term weighing 3.8 kg. Her mother, Clare, is 17 years old and a single parent. A neonatal examination is performed by the neonatal ST1, and Natalie is discharged home at 12 hours of age. She feeds well, and appears to be a content baby. At 6 weeks of age the neonatal examination is missed because Clare is visiting relatives in another part of the country, and the initial immunizations are also delayed by 5 weeks.

Initially Natalie makes normal developmental progress, but is reluctant to crawl and dislikes the prone position. At 13 months she is taken to her GP by her grandmother because of her reluctance to crawl. Natalie moves around the room in a sitting position, pushing herself with her feet.

What other information should you obtain? What is the differential diagnosis?

The GP takes a history, and is told by Natalie's grandmother that Clare had also been reluctant to crawl as a baby. The GP makes a diagnosis of 'bottom-shuffling', and reassures the grandmother. He does not examine Natalie.

At 19 months of age, the GP refers Natalie to a paediatrician with a history of delayed walking.

What does this history suggest?

The paediatrician obtains a more detailed history and discovers that Natalie's father had worn a splint as a baby because of 'clicky hips'. On examination, she finds that Natalie has apparent shortening of her left leg by 2 cm, with reduced abduction and rotation of the hip. A pelvic X-ray is performed (Case Figure 24.1).

What do you think of the X-ray?

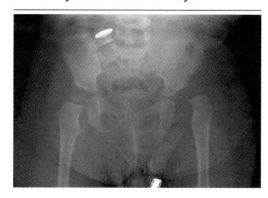

Case Figure 24.1 Natalie's pelvic x-ray

The X-ray reveals a dysplastic left acetabulum with complete dislocation of the left hip. A referral is made to a paediatric orthopaedic surgeon, and Natalie subsequently requires an open reduction of the hip, acetabuloplasty and a femoral shortening osteotomy.

What is the likely long-term prognosis?

A review of the neonatal and maternal notes reveals that the sections for paternal details and history were left blank.

Two years later Natalie's grandmother complains that medical incompetence by the GP and at the hospital led to a delay in the diagnosis with all the resultant adverse sequelae.

Expert opinion

Screening for Developmental Dysplasia of the Hip (DDH) is part of the newborn and 6-weeks physical examination for infants. It is important that this examination is informed by an adequate family history as

Avoiding Errors in Paediatrics, First Edition. Joseph E. Raine, Kate Williams and Jonathan Bonser.
© 2013 John Wiley & Sons, Ltd. Published 2013 by Blackwell Publishing Ltd.

there is a 10-fold increased risk of DDH in the offspring of parents with DDH. In this case, the initial family history in the father was not recorded, the presence of DDH was not identified at the initial examination, and the second hip assessment at 6 weeks was missed. The UK National Screening Committee has set as a standard that 95% of babies with a normal hip examination but 'a family history of a hip problem starting in infancy or as a young child' should have a hip US performed by 6 weeks of age.

In order to perform a neonatal hip examination competently, it is important to understand the anatomy of the neonatal hip, and to practise the examination using clinical simulation with a model such as the 'Baby Hippy' (manufactured by Laerdal). Clinical practice should initially be supervised until it is clear that the technique has been mastered.

All screening procedures have a false negative rate, but an opportunistic hip examination at the time of the delayed immunization might have led to the diagnosis being made. The social history (young, single mother, missed appointments, grandmother (not mother) bringing the baby to clinic) is a clear indicator of added risk in this situation.

'Bottom-shuffling' is common, and can run in families in an autosomal dominant fashion. It is a diagnosis of exclusion, and clinical examination to exclude neuromuscular disorders, cerebral palsy, spinal abnormalities and DDH is important. This opportunity was missed.

The purpose of an early diagnosis of DDH is the early institution of treatment by splintage (e.g. a Pavlik Harness). Natalie was denied this opportunity, required open surgery, and is now at risk of osteoarthritis of the hip as a young adult.

 Legal comment

It seems that the neonatal trainee may have done an inadequate neonatal examination, and failed to diagnose DDH.

The hospital's lawyers will want to take a statement from that doctor. They will want to know why the sections in the maternal and neonatal notes dealing with paternal history were left blank. Did the obstetric staff and the neonatal trainee make any attempt to get those details? Perhaps the mother was unable to provide them?

It is possible that the neonatal trainee will say that he had not had sufficient practice in hip examinations. In that case, his fault lies in not making this clear to his superiors and not ensuring that he was adequately supervised.

However, an expert considering the actions of the neonatal trainee may come to the view that, particularly in the absence of a paternal history, it was not negligent not to make the diagnosis on the first occasion. As stated above all screening procedures have a false negative rate.

Even if the expert view is that the diagnosis should have been made straightaway at birth, it seems very likely that the hospital can pass much of the liability for this case on to the GP practice which did not make a further appointment following the missed 6 week check and which had several opportunities to check again at subsequent appointments for immunizations and when Natalie was 13 months old.

The hospital would argue that if the GP practice had taken those opportunities to redo the examination, as it should have done, then the diagnosis would have been made while it was still possible to treat by splintage, rather than by open surgery. Therefore the GP should take full liability.

The argument would rely on the fact that there is a recognized false negative rate in hip examinations, which puts the GP under a legal duty to re-examine the hip. The failure to examine the patient at 13 months seems particularly indefensible by the GP.

 Key learning points

Specific to the case
1. Family history is an important part of the clinical assessment.
2. Paternal history is often missed or not recorded.
3. Technique is vital when evaluating the newborn hip.
4. If a screening assessment is missed, find out why and attempt to remedy the situation.

General points
1. Pay attention to social risk factors.
2. Remember the absent parent when taking a family history.
3. Absence of documentation does not equate to absence of a risky history.

Further reading and reference

UK National Screening Committee (2008) Newborn and Infant Physical Examination – Standards and Competencies. http://newbornphysical. screening.nhs.uk/getdata.php?id=10639

Case 25 A diabetic girl with a headache

Katie, a 6-year-old girl with a 3-year history of Type 1 diabetes is admitted one afternoon with an 8-hour history of vomiting. Baseline observations are temperature 36.8°C, pulse 106 /min, blood pressure 100/60 mmHg and central capillary refill time (CRT) 4 secs. Katie is seen immediately by the ST1 and ST4 trainees. Her initial venous blood gas shows a pH 7.25, (normal 7.35–7.45) pCO$_2$ 3.4kPa (4.7–6.4 kPa), pO$_2$ 5.4kPa (venous sample), bicarbonate 11mmol/L (22-29 mmol/L), base excess – 10 mmol/L (+2.5 to -2.5 mmol/L) and lactate 3 mmol/L (<2.0 mmol/L). Her bedside finger prick blood glucose is 25 mmol/L (3.5–6.0 mmol/L). The ST1 and ST4 trainees diagnose diabetic ketoacidosis (DKA) and a 20 ml/kg bolus of 0.9% saline is administered intravenously. Katie is estimated to be 10% dehydrated and, in addition to the bolus, is written up for a fluid regime to replace the deficit plus maintenance over the next 48 hours. The National Paediatric DKA protocol is consulted and an insulin infusion is started an hour later at 0.1 units/kg/hour. Her U and Es results are sodium 127 mmol/L (normal 135–145 mmol/L), potassium 4.7 mmol/L (3.5–5.6 mmol/L), urea 4.2 mmo/L (2.5–6.6 mmol/L), creatinine 56 µmol/L (20–80 µmol/L) and laboratory glucose 23.5 mmol/L.

What do you think of the management so far?

When reviewed 4 hours later, Katie is alert and orientated although tired. Her pulse is 90/min, her BP 90/60 mmHg and her CRT 2 secs. However her fluid balance is negative at –350 mls and a repeat venous gas is similar. The bedside blood glucose is 12 mmol/L. The protocol states that a further bolus of 0.9% saline may be needed if there has been no clinical improvement. Senior review is also recommended. The ST4 decides to give her a further bolus of 20 mls/kg 0.9% saline to correct the dehydration.

Would you have done this?

Further electrolytes are sent and the sodium is phoned back as 128 mmol/L and the blood glucose is 11.5 mmol/L.

Would these results alter your management?

The medical team is phoned during handover 4 hours later to say that Katie is complaining of a bad headache and has begun wetting the bed. The nurse accepts a verbal prescription for paracetamol. Half an hour later the night team call the ward and are reassured that Katie is now sleeping and comfortable. They plan to review her later on their night round.

Would you be reassured?

Two hours later the nurses phone to say that Katie is unrousable and has a sluggish pupillary reaction to light. Her blood pressure is 140/100 mmHg and her pulse 56/minute. On examination these findings are confirmed and she is hyperreflexic. A clinical diagnosis of cerebral oedema is made. Hypertonic saline (2.7%) 5 mls/kg is administered iv and the duty consultant and PICU team are summoned. She is ventilated on PICU for 10 days and is left with profound motor and learning disabilities. The parents obtain expert advice and file a lawsuit complaining that the DKA protocol was not followed and that Katie received excess fluids at the outset and during her rehydration.

Expert opinion

Guidelines and protocols are written for a purpose – those for DKA are nationally agreed and have been honed from years of experience. Children and young adults with DKA do not die from shock but usually from

Avoiding Errors in Paediatrics, First Edition. Joseph E. Raine, Kate Williams and Jonathan Bonser.
© 2013 John Wiley & Sons, Ltd. Published 2013 by Blackwell Publishing Ltd.

cerebral oedema which has an incidence of 0.3–1% in DKA. It is unpredictable, more frequent in younger children and newly diagnosed diabetes and has a mortality of approximately 25%. Significant neurological morbidity occurs in 10–26% of survivors. Case-controlled studies have shown that cerebral oedema is probably linked to the overestimation of dehydration and shock, rapid administration of excess crystalloid fluids, too rapid a reduction in blood glucose and, possibly, early use of insulin. The protocol aims to minimize the risks by a slow correction of the metabolic abnormalities.

Katie had mild DKA with no evidence of shock at the outset – her pulse and BP were normal and CRT is a poor sign in DKA as hypocarbia leads to peripheral vasoconstriction. The initial fluid bolus was unnecessary. If used in DKA, boluses should be given in 10 ml/kg aliquots and resuscitation fluids should be subtracted from the 48 hr fluid total. Katie's dehydration was also overestimated – most patients with DKA are only 3–5% dehydrated and no more than 8% should be used in calculations.

Once any shock has been treated it is never urgent to restore physiological normality. At 4 hours Katie was clinically improving and a negative fluid balance is not unusual at this stage. It is crucial to treat the patient and not the figures and Katie did not need the second bolus. The recommended senior review was not sought.

Regular neurological observations are essential in monitoring DKA. Headache and other changes in neurological status such as incontinence should trigger an urgent clinical review because they suggest cerebral oedema and early recognition and management improves outcome. Hypertonic saline or mannitol should be given immediately, maintenance fluids halved and the deficit replaced over 72 hours with close monitoring in a PICU.

Initial dilutional hyponatraemia is common in DKA as the high serum osmolarity drives water from the intracellular to the extracellular space. There is also hypernatruria during the osmotic diuresis. The glucose-corrected serum sodium (Serum Na $+ 0.4 \times$ (Glucose $- 5.5$)) may prove a useful early warning sign of the development of cerebral oedema in DKA. It should rise by about 5 mmol/L over the first 8 hours of therapy. Typically it falls in children who develop late cerebral oedema. This child's initial corrected sodium of 134.2 mmol/L fell to 130.4 mmol/L at 4 hrs.

The final common denominator for all these factors is understanding the risk and minimizing it by paying close attention to detail, making frequent reviews and following the protocol. Any deviation from it should be very carefully considered and discussed with a consultant experienced in DKA. It should also be clearly documented in the notes.

 Legal comment

This is a high-value claim. Katie will require care and support all her life. It will be difficult to defend the actions of the hospital staff. Nonetheless, the lawyers for the NHSLA will want to investigate how the mistake occurred just in case something emerges which might raise an arguable defence.

The crucial question is whether the ST4's decision to administer the second bolus can be justified. If he thought the circumstances justified a departure from the protocol, what were they? Such deviations and the reasons for them should be recorded in the notes at the time. Why did he not get a senior to review the case as the protocol recommended?

Even if the ST4 can give a factual account of events that justifies his decision, the standard of care in the next phase of treatment is highly questionable. It seems that an instructed expert will conclude that the wrong treatment was given (breach of duty) and that, combined with a failure to regularly review, has caused the damage (causation). The claim will probably be settled out of court. The value of the claim will depend on a number of factors, not least of which are Katie's life expectancy and the level of care that she will require. It could easily be several million pounds.

 Key learning points

Specific to the case

1. Children and young people can die from DKA usually due to cerebral oedema.

2. National DKA protocols have been honed over years to minimize this risk and are strongly recommended.

3. Shock and dehydration are often overestimated in DKA leading to the administration of excessive intravenous fluids which may precipitate cerebral oedema.

4. In DKA there is never an urgency to restore normal physiology once any shock has been corrected.

5. Headache or other neurological changes in DKA should trigger an urgent clinical review looking

specifically for raised intracranial pressure due to cerebral oedema.

General points

1. Guidelines and particularly protocols should be adhered to. They have usually been written and refined by experience. Any deviations should be discussed with a consultant and documented in the notes.

2. Senior review of seriously unwell patients is always recommended.

Further reading and references

British Society of Paediatric Endocrinology and Diabetes (2009) BSPED guidelines at: http://www. bsped.org.uk/clinical/docs/DKAGuideline.pdf

Durward A, Ferguson LP, Taylor D *et al.* (2011) The temporal relationship between glucose corrected serum sodium and neurological status in diabetic ketoacidosis. *Arch Dis Child* 96: 50–7.

Case 26 A boy with sickle cell disease and a fever

Lewis, a 9-year-old boy with HbSS sickle cell disease, is brought to the paediatric ambulatory care unit of his local hospital by his aunt on Friday afternoon. He is complaining of limb pain, abdominal pain, headache, fever and vomiting. He has been unwell for 3 days, and initially tried to manage with oral analgesia at home, but today the pain has become much worse. He is usually under the care of the joint paediatric/haematology sickle cell clinic at the hospital. His aunt does not know much about the details of his previous medical history; she is looking after him for a couple of weeks while his parents are in Nigeria. Lewis is due to start a new school term on Monday.

Lewis is alert and orientated, but appears to be in pain. His heart rate is 120/minute, respiratory rate 20/minute, oxygen saturations are 95% in air, and his temperature is 38.4°C. Heart sounds and breath sounds are normal. His abdomen is soft, but slightly tender centrally, and his liver is palpable 3cm below the costal margin. All four limbs appear uncomfortable to move, but there is no focal tenderness, swelling or erythema. There is no meningism. Ear, nose and throat examination is unremarkable.

What would you do now?

Lewis is given oral analgesia (paracetamol, ibuprofen and codeine phosphate) and is encouraged to drink plenty of fluid. Some blood tests are done. By the time the results are back his pain is slightly better:

		Normal
Haemoglobin	7.5 g/dL	11.5–15.5 g/dL
White blood cells	10.5 × 10⁹/L	4–11 × 10⁹/L
Neutrophils	6.9 × 10⁹/L	2–6 × 10⁹/L
Platelets	85 × 10⁹/L	150–400 × 10⁹/L
C-reactive protein	47 mg/L	<6 mg/L
Sodium	132 mmol/L	135–145 mmol/L
Potassium	4.3 mmol/L	3.5–5 mmol/L
Urea	8.0 mmol/L	1.8–6.4 mmol/L
Creatinine	89 μmol/L	27–62 μmol/L

His medical notes arrive and reveal that Lewis has had several previous admissions for painful vaso-occlusive crises, often associated with times of 'stress'. However his last clinic appointment was 4 months ago, and it is noted that his next appointment has been delayed because 'his family are travelling to Nigeria to visit relatives'. His family are Jehovah's Witnesses, but he has never required a blood transfusion and his normal haemoglobin is around 9 g/dL.

Would you do anything different at this point?

Lewis is admitted to the ward, and commenced on iv fluids at 150% maintenance, he is given oral morphine, and blood cultures and a CXR are taken. The CXR shows no lung pathology and he is commenced on iv cefuroxime. He is more comfortable overnight, although he has a spike of fever to 39°C. On the ward round the Registrar notes that Lewis's respiratory rate has increased to 25/minute, but otherwise things have changed little, and she plans to continue current management and repeat the blood tests. However, over the course of the day he develops progressively increasing chest pain, respiratory distress, and hypoxemia, with bibasal shadowing visible on a portable CXR (Case Figure 26.1).

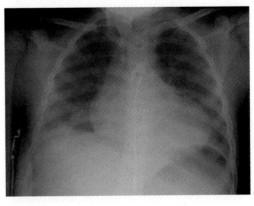

Case Figure 26.1 Lewis's X-ray

Avoiding Errors in Paediatrics, First Edition. Joseph E. Raine, Kate Williams and Jonathan Bonser.
© 2013 John Wiley & Sons, Ltd. Published 2013 by Blackwell Publishing Ltd.

Repeat blood tests show a haemoglobin 6.4 g/dL and the platelet count is now 48×10^9/L. The on-call Consultant manages to telephone Lewis's father in Nigeria to tell him about his son's condition and to discuss the fact that it may be impossible to avoid giving him blood products if he continues to deteriorate. During the course of the conversation Lewis's father asks whether his son has been tested for malaria.

How would you respond?

Lewis goes on to develop a severe sickle chest crisis and requires transfer to a PICU, where he is put on ventilatory support. The consultant again contacts the father in Nigeria and explains that his son needs an urgent exchange transfusion. The father refuses to give his consent. Lewis's aunt grows increasingly concerned as she sees her nephew's condition deteriorate. In discussion with her, it is agreed that he should be given the transfusion. A rapid diagnostic test shows that he has *Plasmodium falciparum* malaria, confirmed by a blood film which shows a parasitaemia of 2%. Lewis is treated with iv quinine. He is discharged from PICU after 5 days. Lewis had travelled to Nigeria with his family for 5 weeks and had returned accompanied by his aunt 8 days before admission. When he had been seen at his last clinic appointment, the family had mentioned that they were going to travel to Nigeria, but antimalarial prophylaxis had not been discussed.

The parents go on to make a formal complaint and sue the hospital stating that Lewis was not diagnosed and treated promptly for malaria, which resulted in him becoming so ill that he needed to have blood transfusions despite being a Jehovah's Witness.

Expert opinion

A travel history is an essential component of history taking for all patients, even when they appear to have an unrelated medical problem. Global travel is now so easy that many children with chronic illnesses can easily travel to locations where they may be exposed to infectious diseases not found in their country of origin. The initial assumption that Lewis simply had a painful sickle cell crisis meant that the admitting doctor did not consider a travel history relevant. Failure to diagnose malaria on admission almost certainly contributed to the development of a severe chest crisis and the need for Lewis to receive blood products. Any traveller returning from a malaria endemic area should be assumed to

have malaria until proven otherwise, ideally with three negative blood films. Whilst the initial blood results for Lewis would be consistent with a bacterial or viral infection triggering this episode of illness, the presence of a low platelet count is a frequent finding in malaria and should have prompted further thought. The medical notes indicated that Lewis's family had mentioned that they were travelling to Nigeria at their last clinic visit (although not specifically that Lewis was going), but no note was made regarding advice on malaria prevention measures. This represents a missed opportunity by the doctor in the clinic, who should really have advised about the risks of malaria if the child did travel, and how to minimize these risks. When the clinic notes were reviewed at the time of the hospital admission there was an additional missed opportunity to realize that Lewis had been to Nigeria. Finally, it appears that the significance of an increase in respiratory rate as a potential indicator of an evolving chest crisis may not have been fully appreciated on the morning following admission.

Legal comment

There are two phases of treatment that need to be considered in this case: when Lewis was seen at the clinic before going to Nigeria; and when he presented with the acute illness.

In the acute phase, he was given a transfusion against his father's wishes. If a child lacks capacity (is not Fraser competent), it is only his parents who can give valid consent for treatment. Or rather, those who have parental responsibility. Could it be argued that the aunt had parental responsibility? In this case, the consultant spoke directly to the father who refused to give his permission for the transfusion. So the answer must be no, unless the father had expressly devolved responsibility to the aunt, which is unlikely. However, this was an emergency situation. In such circumstances, treatment can be given to a child despite the parents' wishes on the basis that the transfusion is in the best interests of the child. Thus, here, the father's wishes could be overridden.

The parents have decided to sue the Trust. Although the acute phase is relevant to their claim (in terms of whether earlier treatment could have prevented Lewis's decline and the need for the transfusion), it is probably what happened before Lewis went to Nigeria that will determine whether the family are successful in pursuing their case. It appears that the staff were told that the boy would be going to Nigeria at his last outpatients appointment. The lawyers will want to know what exactly was said by the family and the clinicians at this consultation. The clinicians should have advised the parents on the need for prophylaxis. If they had, then Lewis would have been far less likely to have fallen ill with malaria and there would have been a far smaller chance of the need for a transfusion. If this can be shown, then the family's claim will be successful and they will be awarded damages.

 Key learning points

Specific to the case

1. Globalization necessitates that a full travel history is always taken, even when the diagnosis seems obvious.

2. Although sickle haemoglobin is partially protective against malaria, patients with sickle cell disease can still get malaria and develop severe disease.

3. Malaria prevention is the duty of all doctors, and those looking after patients with chronic illnesses must ensure that patients planning to travel abroad are fully informed and protected. Essential advice includes: **A**wareness of the risk, mosquito **B**ite avoidance, **C**hemoprophylaxis, and prompt **D**iagnosis of a febrile illness whilst abroad or on return.

4. Travellers visiting friends and relatives abroad are at particularly high risk of travel associated diseases including malaria, because they are least likely to seek medical advice before travelling.

5. Fever in a traveller returning from a malaria endemic area must be assumed to be due to malaria until proven otherwise, even when another diagnosis is present.

6. Clinical features of malaria include: fever, headache, myalgia, abdominal pain and vomiting. Severe manifestations include acidosis, severe anaemia, hypoglycaemia, seizures and coma. Since these features are not unique to malaria, clinical diagnosis of malaria is very unreliable.

7. Thrombocytopenia is often present in malaria.

8. Suspected malaria should be treated as a medical emergency to prevent severe disease.

9. There are published guidelines to assist the management of severe malaria in children in the UK.

General points

1. The need for a travel history should be included in the hospital's paediatric admission guidelines, sickle cell guidelines and/or clerking proformas.

2. The cause of a fever without a focus should always be considered carefully.

3. Blood transfusions may be given to the children of Jehovah's Witnesses without parental consent in the case of an emergency.

Further reading and references

Hagmann S *et al.* (2010) Illness in children after international travel: analysis from the GeoSentinel Surveillance Network. *Pediatrics* 125(5): e1072–80.

Lalloo DG *et al.* (2007) UK malaria treatment guidelines. *J Infect.* 54(2): 111–21.

National Travel Health Network and Centre: http://www.nathnac.org/travel/index.htm

UK Health Protection Agency website: http://www.hpa.nhs.uk/Topics/InfectiousDiseases/InfectionsAZ/Malaria/

Case 27 Negative test results

A 23-year-old South African woman, Della, presents in active labour to a hospital in Wales at 3 am on Saturday morning. This is her second pregnancy and she has gone into spontaneous labour at 34 weeks gestation. She has antenatal notes with her from a hospital in London, which indicate that although she has no significant medical history or obstetric risk factors, she booked late (at 27 weeks) and she has not attended regularly for antenatal care since then. She came to the UK early in this pregnancy and has been staying with different friends around the country. Della delivers a healthy looking female infant, Rose, weighing 2.7 kg, within 20 minutes of arrival. The neonatal ST2 doctor on-call who was at the delivery did not need to resuscitate the infant. However he is concerned that he cannot find a HIV test result in Della's notes. Della reports that she did have the test done, and that she had been told that all her blood tests were fine.

What would you do?

Based on Della's statement the ST2 doctor documents the discussion in her antenatal notes, requesting the obstetric team to follow up Della's HIV serology in the morning. He also adds a note at the bottom of the electronic handover sheet on the computer in the neonatal unit for the doctor on duty the next day to follow-up the result. Unfortunately, the handover sheet on the computer is not saved after the addition of baby Rose's details and is lost when the computer 'crashes' later in the night. The ST2 has a busy night with 26 weeks gestation twins, and is exhausted by the morning. The patient handover the next morning is fragmented because the consultant, registrar and incoming ST2 doctor all arrive at different times. The ST2 doctor on night duty forgets to verbally handover the case to his colleague on duty for the day, and leaves to commence a 7-day holiday. Baby Rose remains well over the next 2 days and breastfeeds well, but is kept on the postnatal ward for observation due to her prematurity. On Monday morning the ST3

doctor covering the postnatal ward checks Rose's notes and discovers that there is no HIV test result, and that the midwives on duty are not aware of any result or additional test having been obtained over the weekend. The ST3 doctor immediately informs her consultant.

What should be done now?

The consultant speaks to Della, counsels her and suggests that a rapid HIV test be performed. The result is positive, and the case is immediately discussed with the regional paediatric HIV specialist, who recommends starting baby Rose on combination therapy as postexposure prophylaxis. Unfortunately, Rose is subsequently found to be HIV infected. Della is depressed, rather than angry, and does not make a complaint because she regards the issue as her fault. However, at the age of 18, her daughter Rose is extremely angry about having HIV and the impact it has on her life, and discovers that she can sue the hospital herself.

Expert opinion

With optimal management the risk of mother to child transmission of HIV should be extremely low, approximately 0.1%. This relies on identification of HIV infected women early in pregnancy, and rigorous implementation of guidelines for their management. A major reason why vertical transmission of HIV continues in the UK is the failure to identify all pregnant women infected with HIV. The Royal College of Obstetricians and Gynaecologists, and the British HIV Association recommend HIV testing for all pregnant women at booking, with timely delivery of results. For all women presenting in labour with an unknown or uncertain HIV status (which would include those with no documented result) a rapid diagnostic test should be performed, which yields a result within 20 minutes. This potentially allows the administration of nevirapine and other antiretrovirals to the mother, delivery by Caesarean section,

Avoiding Errors in Paediatrics, First Edition. Joseph E. Raine, Kate Williams and Jonathan Bonser.
© 2013 John Wiley & Sons, Ltd. Published 2013 by Blackwell Publishing Ltd.

and administration of combination anti-retroviral post-exposure prophylaxis to the newborn within 4 hours of birth, all of which will reduce the risk of vertical transmission. In this case, prematurity, vaginal delivery and breast feeding are all risk factors for mother to child transmission. Failure to perform a rapid diagnostic test for HIV at the time of presentation in labour, and the subsequent failure to verify the maternal HIV status, meant that baby Rose did not have the opportunity to commence anti-retroviral therapy during the optimum time period (within 4 hours) after delivery and that breast feeding was permitted. Although this is the most important error that contributed to the mother to child transmission of HIV in this case, failure to give an adequate handover to the day-time neonatal team and failure to communicate directly and appropriately with the obstetric team probably compounded the problem by limiting the opportunity for other staff to spot the original error.

 Legal comment

Rose will have three years from her 18th birthday to launch the claim before it becomes statute barred. She will first have to get disclosure of her own and her mother's records and then take an expert opinion. That opinion must be based on the standards in place at the time of the incident.

It seems unlikely that the London hospital will be blamed. The results were probably not communicated to the mother, because she was lost to follow-up as she moved around the country visiting friends. The spotlight will therefore be on the hospital in Wales.

The Welsh hospital will probably wish to locate the ST2 doctor to see what he can remember. Although he recorded the need for a HIV test result in the notes, he appears to have then failed to address the matter with the required urgency. He will almost certainly no longer be able to recall the circumstances which prevented him from making an adequate handover.

The hospital's lawyers will also consider whether Rose would have contracted HIV in any event. However, the Expert Opinion states that the failure to commence anti-retroviral therapy within 4 hours of birth and allowing the baby to breast feed were the most important errors that led to the child developing HIV. It seems likely that on balance, Rose would not have acquired HIV, if appropriate treatment had been given. If this is what the instructed experts conclude, then the case will have to be settled.

The hospital's lawyers will, however, argue that some or all of the fault should be placed with Della, the mother, who appears to have given an inaccurate history. They will want to investigate if her negligence contributed to the outcome. This is a matter for negotiation between the lawyers. If the matter cannot be resolved by negotiation, then the judge will have to provide a percentage figure for the reduction in the damages, based on the culpability, if any, of the mother.

 Key learning points

Specific to the case

1. All labour wards should have access to HIV rapid diagnostic tests which can provide a result within 20 minutes.

2. A rapid diagnostic test for HIV should be performed for any woman presenting in labour with an uncertain HIV status. A positive result should be acted on with urgency to maximize the chance of implementing effective interventions before a spontaneous vaginal delivery.

3. Appropriate communication is essential to ensure that neonatal, obstetric and midwifery staff are all aware if a pregnant woman's HIV status is unknown, and all staff should be aware of what needs to be done in the event of a positive test result.

4. If maternal HIV infection is only diagnosed after delivery, the newborn should receive combination anti-retroviral post-exposure prophylaxis as soon as possible (ideally within 4 hours). If treatment is delayed by more than 48–72 hours it is very unlikely to be effective.

5. The planned management of pregnant women with HIV, and their babies, is dependent on many factors, some of the most important being: prior maternal anti-retroviral treatment, maternal viral load at booking and maternal preference for mode of delivery (vaginal or Caesarean section). Often a tailor made treatment plan will be available for the mother and her baby.

6. Changes to the planned management may be necessary if there is: an unsuppressed viral load (>50 copies/ml) at 36 weeks gestation, threatened preterm labour, pre-labour rupture of membranes, or prolonged rupture of membranes during labour. In these circumstances optimal management may be different from that previously planned and expert advice should be sought urgently.

General points

1. Formal, structured handover of patients with freedom from interruptions is essential to prevent communication errors.
2. Hospitals should have policies regarding information that may be stored on electronic handover sheets, and how frequently these should be saved and archived in electronic or paper format.
3. In addition to HIV, it is important for all staff caring for pregnant women and their newborn babies to check results of maternal Hepatitis B and syphilis serology.
4. It should be possible to obtain test results from any hospital in the country at any time of day or night should they be essential for patient care.

Further reading and references

British Medical Association (2004) Safe handover: safe patients. Guidance on clinical handover for clinicians and managers. Available at: http://www.bma.org.uk/images/safehandover_tcm41-20983.pdf (accessed May 2011).

Cunnington A *et al*. Why are some babies still being infected with HIV in the UK? *Adv Exp Med Biol* 659: 57–71.

Royal College of Obstetricians and Gynaecologists (2010) Green-top Guideline No. 39 Management of HIV in Pregnancy. Available at: http://www.rcog.org.uk/files/rcog-corp/GT39HIVPregnancy0610.pdf (accessed May 2011).

Ruiter A de *et al*. (2008) British HIV Association and Children's HIV Association guidelines for the management of HIV infection in pregnant women *HIV Med*. 9(7): 452–502.

Case 28 A bad case of 'flu

During the early phase of an influenza A pandemic, a 10-year-old boy, Michael is brought to the Paediatric ED at his local hospital by his parents. He has a 2-day history of fever, headache, severe myalgia and cough. He has previously been well, except for having problems with recurrent boils over the last 6 months, which have also affected his 7-year-old sister. His observations show a temperature of 38.7°C, heart rate 100/minute, respiratory rate 19/minute, oxygen saturation 97% in air. He is seen by a FY2 doctor, who takes a brief history and performs a basic physical examination which is recorded as normal. She makes a clinical diagnosis of influenza, and requests a nasopharyngeal aspirate (NPA) to confirm the diagnosis.

What would you do?

In keeping with departmental guidelines Michael is prescribed osteltamivir and is discharged home with advice to take antipyretics. Two days later he is brought back to the ED because he has developed vomiting and diarrhoea, intermittently he complains of feeling dizzy and he still has a fever, cough and malaise. Michael's observations show a temperature of 39.5°C, heart rate 135/minute, blood pressure 98/48 mmHg, respiratory rate 35/minute, and oxygen saturation 93% in air. A family friend had recently been treated with osteltamivir and developed vomiting, which he had been told was probably due to the medication, and Michael's parents are rather angry that they were not informed about the possible side effects of the osteltamivir. Michael is seen by the same FY2 who checks the results from the previous attendance and sees that the NPA was positive for Influenza A. She examines him again and notes that he appears flushed, he is not dehydrated, capillary refill time is less than 1 second and his chest has scanty bilateral crepitations.

What would you do now?

Seeing that nausea, vomiting and dizziness are possible side effects of osteltamivir and also symptoms of influenza, the doctor documents a detailed discussion with Michael's family about the possible causes of the current symptoms and advises the parents that they should stop the osteltamivir treatment, continue symptomatic treatment with antipyretics, maintain adequate hydration and return if the symptoms persist for more than 48 hours.

Unfortunately Michael is brought in by ambulance the next morning, having coughed up blood and then collapsed on the floor when his parents tried to get him out of bed. He has signs of shock and requires intubation and massive fluid resuscitation prior to transfer to a PICU. His condition deteriorates due to severe haemorrhagic pneumonia and he becomes impossible to ventilate and has several cardiorespiratory arrests before dying 9 days after his initial presentation. Tracheal aspirates and blood cultures grow methicillin sensitive *Staphylococcus aureus*, which is later found to produce the toxin Panton-Valentine Leukocidin (PVL).

His parents subsequently institute proceedings to try to sue the hospital stating that the diagnosis of pneumonia had been missed and that the delay in treatment resulted in a fatal outcome.

 ## Expert opinion

Bacterial pneumonia is one of the most common complications of influenza in children and can lead to bacteraemia and sepsis. Although this is most frequently caused by *Streptococcus pneumoniae*, influenza is also a risk factor for severe necrotizing pneumonia caused by PVL toxin-producing *Staphylococcus aureus*. Some patients who have carriage of this organism have a history

Avoiding Errors in Paediatrics, First Edition. Joseph E. Raine, Kate Williams and Jonathan Bonser.
© 2013 John Wiley & Sons, Ltd. Published 2013 by Blackwell Publishing Ltd.

of recurrent boils / skin abscesses, as in this case. The initial management of Michael was appropriate with the prescription of osteltamivir being consistent with the guidelines; however, warning signs were missed when he presented the second time. Although the symptoms of fever, diarrhoea, vomiting and 'dizziness' are compatible with influenza, symptoms would normally be starting to improve 4 days after the onset of fever, and especially following osteltamivir treatment. The findings on examination of a flushed child with tachycardia, very rapid capillary refill, tachypnoea and borderline low oxygen saturations are suggestive of sepsis with peripheral vasodilation. Diarrhoea and vomiting are often features of toxin mediated Staphylococcal disease and the 'dizziness' may actually have been due to postural hypotension, a sign of impending circulatory decompensation. The significance of the scanty bilateral crepitations on chest examination was also not appreciated as a sign of developing pneumonia, and was presumably attributed to influenza. Although the junior doctor documented an extensive discussion about osteltamivir and its side effects, she did not appreciate the significance of the clinical findings in this case, and did not discuss the case with a more senior colleague. It is likely that the failure to diagnose signs of a severe infection at an early stage contributed to Michael's death.

 Legal comment

A careful witness statement needs to be taken from the FY2, detailing her findings at each of the two consultations. Can she explain how she interpreted the new findings on the second consultation?

Her statement will then be put to an expert to see if any defence to breach of duty can be made. There should also be an investigation into the likely course of events had the correct diagnosis been made at the second consultation. What treatment would probably have been given and when? Would it have been sufficient to stop the development of the bacterial infection and prevent death?

If, on the balance of probabilities, the infection was already so advanced that treatment would not have been effective and would not have prevented the death, then the hospital could in theory defend this case, because the damage was not the result of any breach of duty.

However, the Trust is likely to wish to settle this case. The parents might expect compensation for the pain and suffering of their son before death, and the statutory bereavement damages of £11,800.

 Key learning points

Specific to the case

1. Bacterial pneumonia is a common complication of influenza. *S. pneumoniae*, *S. aureus* and Group A Streptococci are the most common pathogens.

2. Tachycardia and tachypnoea may be the earliest signs of secondary bacterial pneumonia and/or sepsis in a child with influenza.

3. A child with sepsis may present with 'warm shock' characterized by peripheral vasodilation (capillary refill may be rapid) and a high cardiac output, rather than 'cold shock' where there is peripheral vasoconstriction and a prolonged capillary refill.

4. Panton-Valentine Leukocidin producing *S. aureus* (PVL-SA) is a cause of rapidly progressive severe illness (pneumonia, osteomyelitis and sepsis) in children and young adults, which is frequently not recognized at first contact with health professionals.

5. PVL-SA carriage is also associated with recurrent skin infections, which may affect multiple members of a family.

General points

1. Influenza-like symptoms can be the presenting complaint in life-threatening infections such as meningitis, septicaemia, and malaria. These conditions may be missed without a careful assessment during an influenza pandemic.

2. In an influenza pandemic, a large proportion of patients presenting to hospital services will have microbiologically detectable influenza virus. This finding should not be assumed to be the only cause of their symptoms, or to exclude another coexisting life-threatening diagnosis (e.g. meningococcal disease).

3. Emergency departments should have a system to highlight patients who re-attend.

4. It is good practice for children re-attending hospital with the same illness to be discussed with or seen by a more senior doctor.

Further reading and references

Cunnington A *et al.* (2009) Severe invasive Panton-Valentine Leucocidin positive Staphylococcus aureus infections in children in London, UK. *J Infect* 59(1): 28–36.

Department of Health (2009) Pandemic H1N1 2009 Influenza: Clinical Management Guidelines for Adults and Children. Available at: http://www.dh.gov.uk/en/Publicationsandstatistics/Publications/PublicationsPolicyAndGuidance/DH_107769 (accessed May 2011)

Gillet Y et al. (2002) Association between Staphylococcus aureus strains carrying gene for Panton-Valentine leukocidin and highly lethal necrotising pneumonia in young immunocompetent patients. *Lancet* 2; 359(9308): 753–9.

Case 29 A difficult transfer

Sophie, a 3-year-old girl, attends ED in the evening with a high fever and a history of insect bites. At triage she has a temperature of 40°C, a heart rate of 185/min, CRT of 3 seconds centrally and 4 seconds peripherally, a respiratory rate of 28/min and a SaO2 of 97% in air. She is confused, not recognizing her parents.

Sophie is taken to the resuscitation bay and the paediatric team are asked to come immediately to see her.

The paediatric registrar manages to establish iv access and collects blood for baseline tests, including blood culture and venous gas. The registrar confirms that Sophie is clinically shocked and gives 20 ml/kg of 0.9% saline.

The venous gas shows a pH of 7.19 (normal 7.35–7.45), pCO_2 of 3.5 kPa (4.0–6.5 kPa), BE -7 mmol/L (+2.5 to -2.5 mmol/L) and a lactate of 5 mmol/l (<2 mmol/L). The registrar also fully examines Sophie and finds that the left thigh has an area of firm induration surrounding an insect bite with tracking cellulitis and inguinal lymphadenopathy. He asks the ST1 to prescribe iv ceftriaxone (for sepsis) and iv flucloxacillin (for possible *Staphylococcal* infection).

On reassessment Sophie's heart rate has fallen to 150/min, while the CRT has improved to 2 seconds centrally and 3 seconds peripherally. The registrar gives a second 20 ml/kg bolus and following this Sophie's observations all normalize and she calms down and responds appropriately to her parents.

A plan is made to admit her to the ward with a diagnosis of early sepsis secondary to cellulitis for iv antibiotics and monitoring.

Is this a reasonable course of action?

Approximately 45 minutes after Sophie was last seen by the paediatric team, the ED nurses prepare her for transfer. The cannula inserted by the registrar stops working during the last third of the second antibiotic infusion. This information is communicated to the ward nurses prior to Sophie's transfer to the ward.

During the transfer from the ED to the ward the nurse accompanying Sophie notices that Sophie is becoming confused again. She attempts to take a repeat set of observations, but Sophie is too distressed and routine observations cannot be properly done.

They arrive on the ward just before handover. The ED nurse informs the ward nurse that Sophie is becoming increasingly confused and that the cannula has stopped working. The ED nurse asks the ward nurse to inform the registrar of this. Sophie's mother, informs the nurses that she is going to the canteen to get some food, before it closes.

The ward nurse finds the registrar in the ward office as handover is about to start. She tells the registrar that the cannula has stopped working. The registrar confirms that Sophie has received the majority of the antibiotics before the cannula stopped working. The registrar tells the nurse that the night doctors will site a new cannula after handover.

Should further information have been provided by the nurse?

The doctors finish handover, which takes approximately 40 minutes. After handover the night ST3 goes to site a new cannula.

On entering Sophie's cubicle, he finds that she is apparently asleep. However, when he starts to examine her, he realizes that Sophie is unresponsive. He pulls the crash bell and the night registrar and nursing staff enter the cubicle.

Sophie is found to have a heart rate of 180/min, a CRT of 4 seconds peripherally and centrally, and a respiratory rate of 35/min with a SaO_2 of 94% in air. IV access is secured using an intra-osseous needle and she is given a further 20 ml/kg bolus of 0.9% saline, with no improvement. A full paediatric arrest call is put out this time and a further 20 ml/kg bolus is given.

She continues to deteriorate clinically, despite aggressive fluid resuscitation and inotropes and requires

Avoiding Errors in Paediatrics, First Edition. Joseph E. Raine, Kate Williams and Jonathan Bonser.
© 2013 John Wiley & Sons, Ltd. Published 2013 by Blackwell Publishing Ltd.

intubation and retrieval to the local PICU. However, Sophie goes on to recover and returns to the ward one week later.

The ED nurse subsequently learns what happened to Sophie and fills in an incident form, as the ward nurse failed to act on her concerns that the child was deteriorating on arrival to the ward. The mother goes on to complain that poor monitoring and care of her daughter led to her deterioration and the need for intensive care and that all this could have been avoided with good 'proper' care.

 Expert opinion

The importance of communication errors in critical incidents has been long understood. Early work on this topic was carried out by the aviation industry with the development of Crew Resource Management (CRM) training, which focused on the non-technical skills needed to avoid critical incidents.

This training technique was later adapted by anaesthetists as Anaesthesia Crisis Resource Management (ACRM) and one of the main learning points was the importance of effective communication.

Within paediatrics, research has shown that communication errors are a common component of critical incidents, especially in PICU and during the transfer of critically ill children. There is an increasing use of simulation training to teach ACRM non-technical skills in paediatrics.

In this case, although the initial management of Sophie was entirely appropriate, there was a critical failure of communication. Firstly, between the two nurses and then between the ward nurse and the doctors. While it is impossible to say if there would have been a different outcome had this not happened, it is likely that Sophie would have been dealt with in a calmer fashion with a better outcome for all involved.

 Legal comment

The cannula stopped working during the last third of the second antibiotic infusion. As a result of commu-

nication errors, nothing was done about it for an hour or more. Sophie then collapsed and required aggressive treatment in PICU for a week before she made a complete recovery. If the collapse was due to the cannula problem, which seems likely, then the hospital is liable for any unnecessary pain and suffering caused by the failure to deal promptly with that problem. Sophie's collapse was dramatic, but she covered quickly and well. The damages will not be high. This case highlights a system error, and reinforces the importance of our mantra: communication, communication, communication!

 Key learning points

General points

1. All medical and nursing staff should receive training on the importance of communication errors in critical incidents and on how to minimize them.

2. Handover is a particularly vulnerable time for communication errors. One way to minimize this is to prohibit other high risk activities (e.g. patient transfer) at handover time.

3. Transfer between clinical areas is a high risk activity. The mandatory use of a Paediatric Early Warning (PEW) score prior to a patient leaving one clinical area (e.g. ward, theatres, ED) and again on arrival in a second clinical area can help highlight deteriorating patients.

4. The use of simulation training in clinical areas can help reinforce learning in low frequency, high severity clinical scenarios such as this one.

Further reading and reference

Lim MT *et al.* (2008) A prospective review of adverse events during interhospital transfers of neonates by a dedicated neonatal transfer service. *Pediatr Crit Care Med* 9(3): 289–93.

Case 30 Treatment for tonsillitis

A 3-year-old girl, Lily, is seen at 7 pm in the Paediatric ED having had her second 3 minute typical uncomplicated febrile convulsion. Despite having had appropriate education and reassurance following her first convulsion two months previously, her parents dialled 999. When the ambulance crew arrived Lily had stopped fitting and by the time she reached hospital she was back to normal. The triage nurse documented in the shared medical and nursing notes that for the previous 12 hours Lily had symptoms of an upper respiratory tract infection and apparent difficulty swallowing. Her parents had given her paracetamol at 10 am. She was otherwise healthy, developmentally normal and fully immunized. Her father had had febrile convulsions as a child. Lily was on no regular medication. Her temperature was 39.7°C, pulse 96/minute, central CRT 2 seconds and her airway was patent with no stridor. She is given a dose of paracetamol. An hour later she is reviewed by the ST3 doctor. Her temperature has fallen to 37.5°C, her pulse to 88/minute and she is playing happily. She is flushed but alert with no rash or evidence of meningism. Cardiovascular, respiratory and abdominal examinations are unremarkable. Both eardrums are inflamed and her tonsils are swollen, erythematous and covered in pus. The doctor makes a diagnosis of a febrile convulsion secondary to tonsillitis. She explains this to the parents and they agree that if Lily is still relatively well two hours later than she can go home. In preparation, the doctor writes the discharge letter including a prescription for a 10-day course of penicillin V, noting that Lily had grown group A Streptococcus from a throat swab taken after her first febrile convulsion. The ST3 doctor agrees her management plan with the ST4.

What information is missing?

As per the protocol for dispensing drugs out-of-hours, two nurses check the penicillin so that all is done before the night team arrive. Both medical and nursing staff have their handovers. The department then became extremely busy with a child in the resuscitation room. The nurse now looking after Lily asks one of her junior colleagues to give the parents the antibiotics so that they can leave. The nurse ensures that Lily's parents are happy to go and she is discharged home with safety net advice to return if they are worried.

What is still missing?

An ambulance crew rings an hour later to say that they are on their way back to the hospital having been called when Lily developed severe breathing difficulties 10 minutes after a dose of penicillin. They describe that she has widespread urticaria, lip and tongue swelling, stridor and wheeze. They have given 0.15 mls of 1/1000 intramuscular adrenaline and a 2.5 mg salbutamol nebulizer and are administering 15 litres/min of oxygen via a facemask. In the ED Lily requires a further dose of intramuscular adrenaline, 3 back-to-back salbutamol nebulizers, iv hydrocortisone, chlorpheniramine and a 20 mls/kg fluid bolus. She makes a full recovery.

Her parents write to complain that they had informed the triage nurse that Lily was allergic to penicillin and that she had previously developed a rash and wheeze following this drug. They had explained this the last time they were in and had been prescribed clarithromycin instead. Nobody had asked them about this and they assumed that this was noted in Lily's records. They did not even think to check the bottle of medicine. The paperwork confirms that the triage nurse had clearly documented this history.

Expert opinion

This is a classic example of a systems error as well as there being some individual culpability. Lily's management was exemplary except for the failure of all those involved to communicate and register the penicillin allergy. The triage nurse assumed that her part of the

Avoiding Errors in Paediatrics, First Edition. Joseph E. Raine, Kate Williams and Jonathan Bonser.
© 2013 John Wiley & Sons, Ltd. Published 2013 by Blackwell Publishing Ltd.

notes would be read and that the information would be communicated to others. The ST3 did not read the notes in detail and did not clarify the allergy history herself. Although joint paperwork is generally a positive development, one downside is that doctors do not always take as thorough a history as they would if clerking the patient from scratch. However, a drug and allergies history should always be taken. This should include details of the reaction because there are occasions when a dubious report can be challenged in the safe confines of the hospital, to establish whether the patient is truly allergic. Because of the likelihood that Lily would be discharged after a period of observation, no admission process was completed and no wristband was issued. The latter would have been red instead of white to alert staff to an allergy. Finally, multiple staff were involved, all of whom assumed that someone else had established that Lily was not allergic to penicillin and her parents assumed that the records were already clear from her previous admission.

Inpatient drug charts have a section for allergies that should be checked by ward pharmacists during an admission and when drugs are prescribed to take home, yet numerous national and regional audits have shown that up to 30% remain incomplete. The NHS Patient Safety Federation currently has a work stream entitled 'No Needless Medication Errors' and hospital trust comparative data for allergy documentation is published monthly. Few outpatient or ED prescriptions even include this crucial question. Nor do the written FP10 prescriptions used to get medicines from a local chemist. So the risk is multiplied out of hours or when prescriptions are dispensed without being vetted by a pharmacist. Electronic prescribing may help, but even this is only as good as the data entered. 'Management of Medicines' is one of the 16 core quality and safety standards of the Care Quality Commission, the independent regulator of health and adult social care services in England, against which providers are judged.

Legal comment

It was clearly negligent to administer penicillin to Lily and she suffered an anaphylactic reaction as a result. The mistake was spotted quickly. Appropriate treatment was provided and she made a full recovery. The hospital and doctors should apologize to the family.

If the parents pursue a claim, then damages should be limited to a few hundred pounds, but the full extent of the damages will depend on how severe the reaction was and how long it lasted.

Key learning points

Specific to the case

1. A detailed history of drugs and allergies should always be included in a medical clerking.
2. A history of drug allergy should always be clarified before prescribing or dispensing a drug.

General points

1. Errors are rarely related purely to individual performance. Systems errors are common.
2. There are numerous NHS and government organizations tasked with improving patient safety.
3. Young children rely on their parents to keep them safe and to provide their medical history – this is one of the challenges of paediatric practice.
4. Good communication amongst and between doctors and nurses is pivotal to patient safety.

Further reading and references

Care Quality Commission. www.cqc.org.uk
Patient Safety Federation. www.patientsafetyfederation. nhs.uk

Case 31 Increasing respiratory distress

Adam, a 4-week-old boy born at term, is admitted having had a 20 second 'blue' episode in the GP's evening surgery. He has been breast fed since birth and is gaining weight. Adam's 3-year-old sister has recently had a cold. The day before admission Adam had a runny nose, reduced feeds and fewer wet nappies. The history is otherwise unremarkable. Examination shows a miserable boy with a temperature of 37.4°C, a pulse rate of 160/minute and an oxygen saturation of 89% in air. He has a cough, copious clear secretions and a respiratory rate of 40/minute with mild subcostal and intercostal recession. On auscultation there are widespread fine crackles and expiratory wheezes. The cardiovascular and abdominal examinations are normal.

What is the likeliest diagnosis? What test(s) would you request?

A clinical diagnosis of bronchiolitis is made and a nasopharyngeal aspirate subsequently confirms the cause to be the Respiratory Syncytial Virus (RSV). A CXR is unnecessary at this stage. Adam is administered oxygen via nasal prongs and admitted to the ward for nasogastric feeding and nursing care. Over the next 12 hours his respiratory distress gradually worsens with tracheal tug and increased intercostal and subcostal recession. By the time of the consultant morning ward round Adam is in a headbox requiring 40% oxygen to maintain saturations $\geq$92% and feeds have been stopped due to large gastric aspirates. He has been commenced on iv fluids at 100 mls/kg/day and at the time of the cannula insertion, 2 hours previously, a venous gas had shown a pH 7.28 (normal 7.35–7.45), pCO_2 7.1 kPa (4–6.5 kPa), bicarbonate 23 mmol/L (20–26 mmol/L) and base excess –2 mmol/L (-2.5 to 2.5 mmol/L). A CXR requested due to his clinical deterioration shows patchy atelectasis.

How would you rate the severity of his illness – mild, moderate or severe?

The consultant transfers Adam to the High Dependency Unit, requests 1:1 nursing and close and frequent reviews by the FY2 and ST4 trainees. The possible future need for CPAP is discussed with both staff and parents. Four hours later, Carol, the nurse looking after Adam, asks the FY2 to review the patient because Adam has had several apnoeas and bradycardias lasting up to 30 seconds. His pulse has risen to 190/minute and his oxygen requirement to 60%. The FY2 phones the ST4, Dr Burns, for advice and Dr Burns suggests an ipratropium bromide nebulizer.

Was this a reasonable course of action by the ST4 doctor?

An hour later the nurse, Carol, bleeps Dr Burns to request her to come and review Adam. Carol reports two episodes of apnoea requiring stimulation lasting 90 seconds and that Adam's pulse is now 220/minute. His oxygen saturation cannot be maintained at >87%. Dr. Burns gives a verbal prescription for an adrenaline nebulizer and says that she will attend in about an hour to assess the response.

What would you have done?

Half an hour later the nurse in charge bleeps Dr Burns asking her to attend urgently because the adrenaline has been ineffective and Adam has had two further prolonged apnoeas, desaturating to 54% and requiring intermittent positive pressure ventilation (IPPV) via bag and mask. By the time Dr Burns arrives, the consultant, called by the senior nurse, is already present and bagging the baby. An urgent capillary gas shows a pH 7.08, pCO_2 16.2 kPa, bicarbonate 17 mmol/L and base

Avoiding Errors in Paediatrics, First Edition. Joseph E. Raine, Kate Williams and Jonathan Bonser.
© 2013 John Wiley & Sons, Ltd. Published 2013 by Blackwell Publishing Ltd.

excess – 5 mmol/L. Adam is immediately intubated, ventilated and transferred to a PICU. His course there is complicated by two pneumothoraces and he requires high frequency oscillation. He is an inpatient for a total of 6 weeks and eventually makes a good recovery.

Adam's parents refuse to return to the referring hospital and write a letter of complaint stating that their son had not received appropriate and timely medical care.

 Expert opinion

Bronchiolitis is a common usually self-limiting illness of infancy; 2–3% of infants with RSV positive bronchiolitis are admitted annually with most being managed at home. Typically there is a clinical deterioration over the first 48–72 hrs and babies <2 months may become exhausted and apnoeic. A small proportion of infants need high dependency or intensive care – most respond well to CPAP avoiding the need for intubation. Ventilating such babies has a high complication rate.

There is no evidence that bronchodilators, oral or inhaled steroids have any effect on the clinical course or any important outcomes although they are often tried. There is emerging evidence that adrenaline may be useful. However, the cornerstones of management during a hospital admission are close observation, frequent clinical review and early intervention – all requested by the consultant. This already sick baby's observations showed a continued steady deterioration and the ST4 trainee, Dr Burns, should have gone to see him at the first report of apnoeas and bradycardias. There is a strong possibility that Adam would have responded favourably if CPAP had been started then and avoided the need for intubation. By the time the consultant was called Adam was too sick for this option.

Nursing staff are extremely experienced in caring for children with bronchiolitis and often progress management without medical input. Their request to attend to review such a baby should have been dealt with promptly. They should also be empowered to bypass the trainees and summon the consultant if they have concerns that are not being addressed. Such occasions should be rare.

 Legal comment

Luckily, Adam appears to have made a good recovery. But there were failings in his treatment.

The consultant had requested that the nurses place the child under 1:1 observation and that the FY2 and ST4 trainees should frequently review him. The nurses

appear to have performed their duties. It is the trainees who have been the weak link. As a result, there was a failure to start CPAP.

The expert comments that the trainee should have attended promptly when asked to review Adam. There appears to be a systems failure here. The trainees should appreciate the experience of the nurses and listen to their concerns. In the General Points below, it is suggested that senior nurses should be able to bypass the trainees and contact the consultant, if the trainees do not give adequate attention to their concerns. The fact that the nurses did not do this until a very late stage may indicate that the department is over-hierarchical to the detriment of patient care.

This incident should spark a review of how the trainees, nurses and consultants all interact.

 Key learning points

Specific to the case
1. High-risk babies with bronchiolitis require frequent clinical review and those <2 months of age are at particular risk of becoming exhausted and apnoeic.
2. Early CPAP may prevent the need for intubation and ventilation which carries considerable morbidity.

General points
1. Paediatric nurses are usually very experienced at caring for children. Their request for a review should not be delayed or refused.
2. If the severity of a situation is not clear from a phone conversation or a handover from an inexperienced junior, it is safest to review the patient immediately.
3. Senior nurses should be empowered to bypass the trainees and summon the consultant if they have concerns that are not being addressed.
4. Recognizing which children are at greater risk of complications from common disorders and therefore need frequent reviews is a crucial skill for paediatricians to acquire.

Further reading and references

Bush A, Thomson A (2007) Acute bronchiolitis. *BMJ* 335: 1037–41.

Hartling L *et al.* (2011) Steroids and bronchodilators for acute bronchiolitis in the first two years of life: systematic review and meta-analysis. *BMJ* 342: d1714.

Case 32 A feverish girl with poor feeding

A 10-month-old female infant, Elena, is brought to the ED with a history of fever for 1 day, measured at 39°C. She has been unwell with poor feeding, but with no symptoms of any specific disease. At triage Elena is afebrile (36°C), with a heart rate of 185/min, CRT of < 2 seconds centrally and peripherally, respiratory rate of 30/min and SaO$_2$ of 99% in air.

She is seen directly by the paediatric ST2. Her observations remain unchanged and the ST2 can find no focus for any infection. Elena remains afebrile.

The ST2 discusses Elena with the paediatric registrar. They decide to admit the child to the ward for observation and to carry out a partial septic screen; blood tests (including CRP and blood cultures), a CXR and a clean catch urine sample. The blood tests and CXR are performed before Elena leaves the ED. An attempt is made at iv access but fails and a decision is taken not to make a second attempt. Elena is transferred to the ward where she is placed in a side room, and her mother is asked to collect a urine sample.

Is this a reasonable course of action?

The night team arrive and Elena is handed over as being generally well with a history of reported fever, but no signs on examination. The CXR is reviewed and is normal. The blood tests are still awaited.

At nursing handover it is reported that a urine sample hasn't been collected and a decision is taken to try again in the morning. The nurses have no plan from the doctors as to the frequency of observations and a plan is made for routine 4 hourly observations.

Is this an appropriate course of action?

At midnight, Elena is found to be cold with a temperature of 35.5°C, heart rate 190/min and cool feet. The window to the room is open and the low temperature is thought to be environmental. The window is closed and a blanket is placed on her. The doctors are not contacted.

At 04.00, Elena is still cold and the temperature is unchanged at 35.5°C, despite the earlier measures. The night ST2, Dr Edmunds, is contacted. He is in ED with a combative alcohol-intoxicated teenager and does not feel he can leave. He reviews Elena's blood results and is reassured by a CRP of 8 mg/L (normal<6 mg/L) and a total WCC of 3.0 × 10^9/L (4.5–15 × 10^9/L). He advises the nursing staff that he will come and review her as soon as he is able, but that she is unlikely to have a significant illness. He asks the nursing staff to call the night time registrar, Dr Stark.

Dr Stark is called but is busy on the neonatal unit and also advises the nursing staff that she will review the child as soon as she is able to.

Is this a reasonable course of action?

At 05.00, Dr Edmunds reviews Elena. He finds that her temperature is now only 35.0°C, she is cold to the knees and elbows with a peripheral CRT of 5 seconds and a heart rate of 210/min. The respiratory rate is now 40/min, but the SaO$_2$ remains 99% in air.

Dr Edmunds, fast bleeps the registrar and then tries to gain iv access. When Dr Stark arrives she inserts an intra-osseous needle and puts out a full paediatric cardiac arrest call. Elena is given two 20 ml/kg boluses of 0.9% saline, but does not respond. Two further 20 ml/kg boluses are given and the heart rate comes down to 170/min and she becomes warm to the ankles and wrists. However, the respiratory rate rises to 50/min and she requires 10 L/min of O$_2$ to maintain a normal SaO$_2$.

After discussion with the on-call paediatric and anaesthetic consultants, Elena is electively intubated and the local retrieval team is asked to transfer her to a PICU. Two further 20 ml/kg boluses are required to maintain perfusion before she leaves for PICU and broad spectrum antibiotics are started

Avoiding Errors in Paediatrics, First Edition. Joseph E. Raine, Kate Williams and Jonathan Bonser.
© 2013 John Wiley & Sons, Ltd. Published 2013 by Blackwell Publishing Ltd.

On PICU Elena requires ventilation for three days. A catheter urine sample and the blood culture grow a coliform, and she is subsequently found to have a horseshoe kidney and vescico-ureteric reflux. She goes on to make a full recovery.

The PICU asks the local hospital to investigate why Elena deteriorated so markedly in hospital.

Expert opinion

Paediatric septicaemia results from the spread of microorganisms into the bloodstream, triggering a systemic inflammatory response syndrome (SIRS). It can be caused by many different organisms, but the end result is a picture of fever or hypothermia, with a tachycardia and tachyopnea.

Early signs of paediatric sepsis are often subtle, for example a mildly elevated heart rate, and any patient with an unexplained tachycardia needs to be monitored closely for signs of deterioration.

Hypothermia in sepsis is a well recognized finding and hypothermia in a child who has been previously febrile should not be ignored.

In this case the initial plan to admit for observation is valid, but in these cases, children must be observed regularly (e.g. 1 hourly observation). If a change in parameters is then found the child should be re-examined.

The ST2, Dr Edmunds, was also falsely reassured by the 'normal' inflammatory markers (often normal in early sepsis) and did not consider obtaining a catheter specimen urine or a suprapubic aspirate when Elena was still well. In fact, a low WCC can also be a sign of sepsis (this is thought to be related to a consumptive phenomenon).

The large volumes of fluid required by Elena to maintain perfusion are not unusual in paediatric sepsis related shock. The inevitable consequence of pulmonary oedema that follows large volume resuscitation should be anticipated and early elective intubation should always be considered.

Although Elena suffered no permanent harm, the care provided by the local hospital was substandard.

Legal comment

Luckily Elena suffered no permanent harm. The parents have made no formal complaint. However, there are clearly lessons to be learnt from the incident, to prevent the same errors being repeated. Neither the nurses, nor the ST2 were sufficiently aware of the potential significance of the hypothermia. Next time, the outcome may not be so fortunate.

There were individual failings in Elena's treatment and the systems in place do not appear to be effective. As indicated in the General Points below, when a child is admitted for observation, the nursing staff should be told how often they are to be observed.

Key learning points

Specific to the case

1. Hypothermia is as important (if not more important) an indicator of sepsis as a high fever.
2. An unexplained tachycardia should never be ignored.
3. A low WCC in the presence of a febrile illness may be a marker of sepsis.

General points

1. When admitting a child for observation it is important to clarify with the nursing staff the frequency of observations.
2. The use of Paediatric Early Warning (PEW) scores can help nursing staff know when to request a medical review of a sick child.

Further reading and references

Goldstein B *et al.* (2005) International pediatric sepsis consensus: Definitions for sepsis and organ dysfunction in pediatrics. *Pediatr Crit Care Med* 6(1): 2–8.

Santhanam S *et al.* (2011) Pediatric Sepsis www.emedicine.medscape.com/article/972559-overview

Case 33 An infant with a swollen face

A 9-month-old Chinese boy, Jiang, is taken to the GP by his mother because he has a swollen, bruised left cheek. His mother, Lien, speaks no English but the GP is Chinese speaking. Lien says that Jiang crawls and that he hit the left side of his head on a coffee table the previous day. She says he cried but did not lose consciousness.

On examination there is extensive swelling over the left zygoma which is tender and a red bruise over Jiang's left upper eyelid.

He is sent to the hospital for a X-ray of the zygoma and Lien is told to return to the GP in 2 days time.

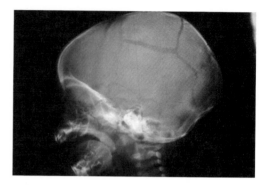

Case Figure 33.1 Jiang's x-ray demonstrating the long parietal skull fracture

What do you think of the GP's management?

Lien, does not return to the GP as planned and the GP does not take any further action until he receives the X-ray report a week later. The report states that there is a possible skull fracture and advises that further X-rays be performed. The GP attempts to contact Lien but her mobile phone is switched off and two days later he has still not been able to contact her.

What should the GP do now?

The GP contacts the Health Visitor who visits Lien and tells her to go to hospital. Jiang returns to hospital and is seen by an ED FY2 doctor who is not aware of the details of the case but knows that a full set of skull X-rays is required. These show a long parietal skull fracture (Case Figure 33.1).

What should the ED FY2 doctor do now?

Jiang is admitted to the paediatric ward for a further assessment. A CT brain scan is performed as the NICE Guideline on Head Injuries recommends a CT brain scan in all cases of head injury when there is a clinical suspicion of nonaccidental injury.

Via a Chinese interpreter the following history is obtained. On the day of the fall, Lien, his mother, was in the same room but had her back turned. She heard him fall and thought that he had been pulling himself up to stand and had then fallen, hitting the left side of his face on the edge of the coffee table. He cried for a minute and then seemed to be back to normal. Two hours later his face became swollen. She decided not to go to the doctor that evening as she knew that the Chinese speaking doctor would not be in the surgery until the next morning. That night Jiang was fretful and seemed uncomfortable when lying on his left side. The following day he seemed generally fine but the swelling was more marked.

Avoiding Errors in Paediatrics, First Edition. Joseph E. Raine, Kate Williams and Jonathan Bonser.
© 2013 John Wiley & Sons, Ltd. Published 2013 by Blackwell Publishing Ltd.

The boy lives with Lien and his 4-year-old sister. Lien says that her husband ran off with another woman when she was pregnant with the boy and that there has been no further contact. She often leaves the children with a female friend and they had been with her the day before the reported incident.

A full examination is performed and no other signs of injury are detected.

The CT scan is normal apart from the skull fracture. When Lien is told about the skull fracture she becomes upset, worried and concerned. She goes very pale and asks whether this will affect his future development. The paediatric registrar feels that the injury is consistent with the history and that the mother's affect is appropriate and so Jiang is allowed home the next day with an appointment to return to clinic five days later. The following day the X-rays are reviewed by a consultant paediatric radiologist who contacts the responsible consultant paediatrician to say that the skull fracture is extensive, branching, crosses a suture and involves the occiput and that nonaccidental injury should be strongly considered.

What should the consultant paediatrician do now?

Jiang is readmitted and a skeletal survey is performed which shows a buckle fracture of the left distal radius. Lien is told about this fracture but can offer no explanation for it. Fundoscopy is performed by a consultant ophthalmologist and shows no abnormality. A strategy meeting is held and a Section 47 (child protection) investigation is commenced by Children's Social Care (CSC).

The police inform CSC that the father is in prison. He was convicted of serious violent crimes and has been sentenced to 10 years imprisonment. Lien is fully aware of this and had attended the trial. She is interviewed by the police and gives a completely different account of the events leading up to her taking the boy to the GP. She admits lying to the doctors about the fall against the coffee table and says that the injury happened when the boy was in the care of her friend. The sister discloses that their mother hit her with a shoe leaving red marks on her body.

Both children are taken into care. Lien is charged with grievous bodily harm to Jiang but is not convicted because the cause of his injuries cannot be established beyond reasonable doubt.

 Expert opinion

The GP was concerned that Jiang might have a fractured zygoma. This would be an unusual injury for a child of this age. A detailed history should have been taken to explore all the possible ways in which such an injury could have occurred and to elucidate who had been in contact with the child in the preceding days when the injury might have happened. The extensive swelling was probably serious enough to warrant immediate referral to a paediatrician rather than just sending Jiang for a X-ray. The follow-up arrangements were not robust enough for a young child with a serious injury. When Jiang was not brought back for follow-up, alarm bells should have rung. The GP could also have done a home visit, contacted CSC or contacted the police. He could have sought advice from a consultant paediatrician or the named doctor or nurse for child protection. When things began to go wrong the GP should have contacted a paediatric registrar or consultant so that Jiang was not dealt with by a junior ED doctor who was not in possession of all the relevant information. Good communication is always essential in managing cases of possible deliberate harm.

 Legal comment

It is difficult to secure a conviction for child abuse without firm evidence which meets the criminal standard of proof which is 'beyond reasonable doubt'. In this case, it may be that no-one will ever be convicted for the injury done to Jiang.

We are told that Jiang and his sister have been taken into care. There will now be civil proceedings in the family courts to determine where they should live in the future. The courts are encouraged to deal with matters within a 'timetable for the child', ideally 40 weeks, but that may prove difficult to achieve if his mother, Lien, challenges the plans which are put forward. In practice, the proceedings could take a year or so to reach a conclusion.

What are their prospects of being restored to Lien? Much depends on her approach to the enquiries. Although she has lied to the GP, and then to the hospital doctors, she did then admit her lies to the police. The cultural pressures on her will be taken into consideration, but generally, the more cooperative she is in the future, the better the prospects of the family being eventually reunited.

Enquiries will be made into Lien's circumstances to establish whether it is in her children's best interests to return to her. If the conclusion is that it is not, the children are young enough to have a prospect of finding adoptive parents.

As for the GP in this case, he is heavily criticized by the expert for not responding quickly enough. In the hospital too there were delays, for example in establishing the extent of the skull fracture and that there was also a fractured arm.

These are matters which should certainly be investigated by the hospital and/or the GP's PCT. That investigation will hopefully lead to improved communication and to heightened awareness. It is possible that the investigation report will suggest that the failings by individuals are potential disciplinary matters and consideration should be given to reporting them to the GMC.

 Key learning points

Specific to the case

1. The child's developmental stage is important. Jiang at the age of nine months was crawling and pulling himself up to stand but was not yet ambulant. It is therefore very unlikely that he would have sustained a skull fracture, particularly a complex one, from a low velocity domestic fall and statistically this increases the likelihood that the injury was nonaccidental.

2. This case should have been brought to the attention of a consultant paediatrician as soon as it was realized that there was a delay in presentation, a complex skull fracture and an inadequate explanation for how the fracture had occurred.

3. Worrying features of a skull fracture which raise the likelihood of nonaccidental injury include multiple or complex fractures (e.g. branching, crossing a suture, more than one bone involved, occipital fracture(s), maximum fracture width >3 mm).

4. This case demonstrates the importance of combined information and opinions from multiple agencies. In this case health agencies and the police all had important information which CSC needed to be aware of.

General points

1. If a GP has the slightest suspicion of nonaccidental injury, he should refer immediately to a paediatrician, especially if the child is young.

2. If the parent/carer does not speak English it is imperative to have an interpreter for all interviews. Even with an interpreter it can be difficult to understand the nuances of a case as sometimes individual words do not have direct translations.

3. Paediatricians are trained to 'listen to the mother' and to 'believe the parents'. It can be extremely difficult to spot the mother who is lying, covering up or deliberately deceiving professionals, especially when there are language and cultural barriers.

4. X-rays taken in cases of possible nonaccidental injury must be reviewed by a consultant radiologist with a special interest in paediatrics and experience in child abuse cases. Ideally, there should be a face to face discussion, with the images available, between the consultant paediatrician and the consultant radiologist in all such cases.

5. The Welsh Child Protection Systematic Review Group provides systematic reviews defining the evidence base for the recognition and investigation of physical child abuse and neglect including fractures and skull fractures.

Further reading and references

Hobbs CJ (1984) Skull fracture and the diagnosis of abuse. *Arch Dis Child* 59: 246–52; doi:10.1136/adc.59.3.246

Hobbs CJ, Wynne JM, Hanks H (1993) *Child Abuse and Neglect: A Clinician's Handbook.* Edinburgh: Churchill Livingstone.

NICE Clinical Guideline (2007) Head Injury. Triage, assessment, investigation and early management of head injury in infants, children and adults. www.nice.org.uk/CG56

Welsh Child Protection Systematic Review Group. www.core-info.cf.ac.uk/

Case 34 Starting a new treatment

Sanna, a 14-year-old girl with severe Crohn's disease, who has relapsed after multiple courses of corticosteroids and azathioprine, is evaluated for treatment with the anti-Tumour Necrosis Factor (TNF) agent, infliximab.

What risks of biological agents should be discussed with the girl and her family?

Before commencing treatment Sanna's vaccination status and the presence of anti-Varicella antibodies are confirmed and she has a tuberculin skin test and a CXR. She had received neonatal BCG (and has a scar over her left deltoid) because her parents are originally from Pakistan. The tuberculin skin test shows no induration at 48 hours, and the ST2 doctor records 'negative tuberculin test' in Sanna's notes. The CXR is normal.

How would you interpret these results?

Sanna receives 3 infusions of infliximab over the next 6 weeks and has a substantial improvement in her condition. Five weeks later she presents to her local paediatric unit complaining of fever and is seen by a ST1. She has felt increasingly unwell over the last week, with intermittent fever, loss of appetite, abdominal pain, poor sleep, vomiting, and her parents report that she has become extremely withdrawn. On examination, Sanna has lost 2 kg over the last week 5 weeks, she has a temperature of 38.4°C and mild central abdominal tenderness without guarding or rebound tenderness. Otherwise cardiovascular, respiratory, abdominal and ear, nose and throat examinations are unremarkable.

What causes should be considered for this illness?

After discussion with the registrar, Sanna is admitted to the paediatric ward, with a tentative diagnosis of a relapse of Crohn's disease and a differential of sepsis or viral gastroenteritis. She has some routine blood tests including blood cultures. These reveal:

	Normal
Hb 9.6g/dL	12–15 g/dL
WBC 12.3 × 10^9/L	4.5–13 × 10^9/L
Neutrophils 6.8 × 10^9/L	1.5–6 × 10^9/L
Platelets 227 × 10^9/L	150–400 × 10^9/L
CRP 48 mg/L	<6 mg/L
Albumin 26 g/L	37–50 g/L

How would you manage this girl?

Transfer to the regional referral centre is not possible due to a bed shortage, but Sanna's case is discussed with the on-call paediatric gastroenterology registrar, Dr Brennan. Following Dr Brennan's advice, a CXR is performed to rule out tuberculosis, blood, urine and stool cultures are taken, intravenous ceftriaxone and metronidazole are commenced, and abdominal and pelvic USs are performed to exclude an abscess. Over the next five days Sanna continues to have intermittent fevers but all her cultures are negative and the CXR is normal. She is extremely withdrawn and starts to become confused and drowsy with neck stiffness on examination. At this stage an urgent CT scan of her head is performed which shows basal meningeal enhancement and moderate hydrocephalus.

What is the likely diagnosis and what would you do now?

In view of the radiological features, a diagnosis of tuberculous meningitis is suggested by the radiologist. A LP is not performed due to Sanna's fluctuating conscious level. She goes on to have a complicated course with several acute neurological deteriorations requiring

Avoiding Errors in Paediatrics, First Edition. Joseph E. Raine, Kate Williams and Jonathan Bonser.
© 2013 John Wiley & Sons, Ltd. Published 2013 by Blackwell Publishing Ltd.

admission to PICU and her parents claim that she subsequently seems to have a reduced intellectual performance. For this reason they sue the hospitals involved, stating that Sanna was not properly assessed for risk of tuberculosis and that the diagnosis was delayed.

 Expert opinion

Although pulmonary disease is the most common manifestation of tuberculosis, extrathoracic and disseminated disease can occur without chest signs, particularly in infants and the immunocompromised. Tuberculous meningitis (TBM) often causes vague symptoms initially such as fever, weight loss and anorexia, and classical signs of meningism only evolve later. For this reason TBM is frequently diagnosed late, when there is already hydrocephalus and an increased risk of neurological sequelae. To prevent this it is particularly important to identify risk factors for tuberculosis and to have a low threshold for investigating early in a child with suggestive symptoms. There is increasing use of anticytokine biological agents, many of which increase the risk of sepsis, and the risk of reactivation of latent tuberculosis is particularly increased by anti-TNF agents. Prior to commencing treatment with Infliximab, evaluation for latent tuberculosis is recommended. Unfortunately immunosuppression, prolonged illness and malnutrition can all contribute to a falsely negative tuberculin skin test. In this case it is highly suspicious that there was no response to tuberculin in a child who had previously received BCG. This suggests that either Sanna was anergic due to immunosuppression or that the tuberculin was administered incorrectly; in either case the test becomes invalid. Here, the significance of the unreactive tuberculin test was not realized, and Sanna was managed as if there was no risk of reactivation of latent tuberculosis. Ideally there should have been an additional risk assessment from a detailed history of possible tuberculosis exposure, an interferon-gamma release assay, and either treatment for latent tuberculosis or very careful observation and education of the family about the risk. When Sanna developed symptoms, the reliance on a CXR to rule out tuberculosis neglected the fact that reactivation in immunosuppressed patients may not manifest as pulmonary disease. Failure to consider this possibility led to a delay in the diagnosis and treatment of TBM, and may have contributed to the outcome. The most common neurological sequelae of TBM include intellectual impairment and motor deficits.

 Legal comment

The actions of the ST2 doctor who conducted the tuberculin skin test need to be considered. It seems possible that the false negative result was due to his not administering the test correctly. If so, that would clearly be negligent.

However, if he did administer the test correctly, is there a responsible body of medical opinion which would hold that it was acceptable for him (and the doctors who then administered the infliximab) to rely on that test result? Were the circumstances such that the skin test might responsibly be thought to be a sufficient evaluation for latent tuberculosis?

If not, then there appears to have been a breach of duty at that point. Even if there was no breach of duty, the actions of the registrar, Dr Brennan, still need to be considered. Is there a responsible body of medical opinion which would hold that it was acceptable in the circumstances to rely on a CXR to rule out tuberculosis? If not, then there is liability for the consequence of that failure.

If the Expert Opinion is that there has been a breach of duty, then the question is, what were the consequences of that breach? If there is intellectual impairment, then it seems likely to be linked to the TBM. Would earlier treatment have made a difference? If the answer is 'probably yes', then Sanna will need to be assessed by a neurologist some years later, when the full extent of the disability and its likely impact become clear. The case may therefore take some time to conclude. It is, of course, a potentially costly case.

 Key learning points

Specific to the case

1. A tuberculin skin test (Mantoux test) can give a false negative result in children who are malnourished or immunosuppressed by serious illness (it may even occur in children who have a prolonged illness due to tuberculosis), immunodeficiency, or immunosuppressive medications. Immunological tests (interferon gamma release assays) may have better sensitivity for diagnosis of latent tuberculosis and should be used in addition to skin testing.

2. Documentation of the exact result (millimetres of induration), rather than positive or negative, is

very important for the subsequent interpretation of the tuberculin test.

3. Children receiving immunosuppressive treatments are vulnerable to severe, opportunistic and unusual infections and to reactivation of latent infections, all of which may present in an unusual way.

4. The initial symptoms of tuberculous meningitis (TBM) can be very nonspecific. A high index of suspicion is necessary in those at risk.

5. TBM can occur without pulmonary involvement: a normal chest radiograph does not exclude tuberculosis.

General points

1. BCG vaccination is most protective against TBM and disseminated tuberculosis in infants. The protective effect of BCG against pulmonary tuberculosis is less, with an enormous range of estimates of efficacy (from 0 to 80%) depending on geographical setting and strain of vaccine used.

2. Treatment for latent tuberculosis carries a small risk of serious side effects, principally hepatotoxicity.

3. Good communication between subspecialist services and local paediatric services is very important for children with complex medical problems who may present to their local hospital with complications of their underlying condition or its treatment. Ideally such problems should be anticipated, and guidance on appropriate management provided, and local hospitals should maintain frequent contact with the specialist centre if these children are admitted.

Further reading and references

Department of Health (2007) Immunisation against infectious disease – 'The Green Book'. Tuberculosis, Chapter 32. Available at http://www.dh. gov.uk/en/Publicationsandstatistics/Publications/ PublicationsPolicyAndGuidance/DH_079917 (accessed May 2011)

National Institute for Health and Clinical Excellence (2011) Tuberculosis. Clinical diagnosis and management of tuberculosis and measures for its prevention and control. http://www. nice.org.uk/guidance/CG117 (accessed May 2011)

Theis VS, Rhodes JM (2008) Review article: minimizing tuberculosis during anti-tumour necrosis factor-alpha treatment of inflammatory bowel disease. *Aliment Pharmacol Ther* 27(1): 19–30.

van Well GT *et al.* (2009) Twenty years of pediatric tuberculous meningitis: a retrospective cohort study in the western cape of South Africa. *Pediatrics* 123(1): e1–8.

Case 35 The importance of interpretation

A 4-month-old Pakistani infant, Arif, presents to the ED with a 24-hour history of abnormal movements. One of the episodes is witnessed by the triage nurse who feels that Arif is having a tonic-clonic fit with loss of consciousness. That episode lasts for 4 minutes but there have been five other episodes in the past 24 hours, the longest being for 15 minutes. Arif is fully breast fed and has not been weaned yet. There is no other relevant medical history.

Arif has a temperature of 37.1°C, a flat fontanelle and no rash. The paediatric ST1 can elicit no abnormal signs. The blood glucose is normal at 5.1mmol/L. Following discussion with the registrar, who is primarily concerned about the possibility of meningitis, a FBC, CRP, U and E's, bone chemistry, LFTs, blood cultures, urine culture and a LP are performed and iv ceftriaxone and aciclovir are administered.

The results are as follows:

		Normal
Hb	9.2 g/dL	9.0–13.0 g/dL
WBC	17.2 × 10⁹/L	4.5–15.0 × 10⁹/L
Neutrophils	9.1 × 10⁹/L	1.5-8.0 × 10⁹/L
Platelets	362 × 10⁹/L	150–400 × 10⁹/L
U and E's	Normal	
Calcium	1.52 mmol/L	2.20–2.75 mmol/L
Phosphate	2.62 mmol/L	1.30–2.10 mmol/L
ALP	878 U/L	145–420 U/L
LFTs	Normal	
CRP	1 mg/L	<6 mg/L
CSF		
WBC	4 × 10⁶/L	<5 × 10⁶/L
RBC	2 × 10⁶/L	0–2 × 10⁶/L
Gram stain	Negative	
Protein	0.38 g/L	0.20–0.40 g/L
Glucose	3.6 mmol/L	2.8–4.4 mmol/L
Urine dipstick	Negative	

Overnight Arif has 3 more fits and requires iv lorazepam on 2 occasions. He remains apyrexial.

What is your opinion of the investigation results and the treatment to date?

At the 8.30 am handover the consultant notes the low calcium that is documented in the handover sheet and asks the ST1 about the low calcium and how it could relate to the fitting. After a pause, the ST1 states that he did notice that it was low but that he didn't think that it was low enough to cause a fit. The result had not been discussed with the registrar.

What do you think the likely diagnosis is and which further investigations would you do?

A diagnosis of rickets with hypocalcaemic fits is made. A blood sample is immediately obtained for vitamin D, parathyroid hormone levels, Mg and repeat bone chemistry and an urgent blood gas analysis (which also measures a number of electrolytes) is performed which shows the ionized calcium to be low. A ferritin level and a haemoglobinopathy screen are also performed and a wrist X-ray is also ordered.

What treatment would you administer?

IV calcium gluconate is administered. Oral calcium and vitamin D are also prescribed. The wrist X-ray provides further confirmation of the rickets. The calcium and phosphate levels normalize and Arif stops fitting. The ceftriaxone and aciclovir are stopped.

The ferritin level is also low and Arif is commenced on a 3-month course of iron.

He is discharged with a 3-month course of vitamin D and with dietary advice.

What else should be done?

The mother who is dark skinned, mostly covered in traditional dress and a vegetarian, is referred to her GP

Avoiding Errors in Paediatrics, First Edition. Joseph E. Raine, Kate Williams and Jonathan Bonser.
© 2013 John Wiley & Sons, Ltd. Published 2013 by Blackwell Publishing Ltd.

who diagnoses her as also having vitamin D deficient rickets. Arif is well and thriving on subsequent clinic follow-up.

The mother complains stating that he had unnecessary investigations, unnecessary drugs and multiple fits due to the delay in diagnosis.

 Expert opinion

Hypocalcaemic fits in infancy secondary to rickets are rare, but this possibility should nevertheless have been on the differential diagnosis list in Arif. Whether Arif, who was afebrile and had no signs of meningitis such as a bulging fontanelle, should have had a LP and iv antimicrobials immediately, or whether he should have been observed pending the preliminary investigation results is debateable. It would be reasonable to do a LP and give antimicrobials on the grounds that meningitis and encephalitis can be difficult to diagnose in infants, they are a common cause of fits in infants and early treatment for these conditions is very important. Treatment can then be stopped if the patient's condition and the investigation results suggest an alternative diagnosis.

Having received the above results, which should have been obtained urgently, the diagnosis should have been reviewed. One of the advantages of having a patient in hospital is that they can be observed carefully and repeatedly reviewed. The slightly raised blood WBC count is probably secondary to the fitting. The results exclude meningitis and it would be highly unusual to have encephalitis with a normal CSF result. The normal urine dipstick suggests that a urine infection is very unlikely and Arif does not have the features of the two other common serious infections, pneumonia and septicaemia. A significant infection is therefore unlikely.

Not only is it the responsibility of the doctor ordering the investigations to check the results (or to ask a colleague to do so) but they must also act on them. If there is uncertainty about a result then it should be discussed with a more senior doctor. The registrar's supervision of the ST1 should also be investigated.

Many doctors would use their initiative and use search engines such as Google to look up hypocalcaemia in infants to discover more about this condition. Diagnosis and treatment should have been speedier but fortunately Arif does not seem to have sustained any long-term harm from his repeated fits.

 Legal comment

According to the Expert Opinion, it was acceptable to do a LP, but Arif may have been spared the three fits and

the iv lorazepam during the night, if an earlier diagnosis had been made. The paediatric ST1 failed to act on the low calcium results. This is unacceptable. The hospital should apologize unreservedly for the error that the ST1 made and should consider whether the ST1 needs further training in view of his mistake.

 Key learning points

Specific to the case

1. The best source of vitamin D is sunlight. Vitamin D is produced endogenously when ultraviolet rays from sunlight strike the skin and trigger vitamin D synthesis. Having dark skin is a risk factor for rickets as dark skinned individuals produce less vitamin D in response to sunlight. Oily fish is the best dietary source of vitamin D and margarine and cereals are often supplemented with vitamin D.

2. Infantile rickets with hypocalcaemic fits is known to occur in primarily breast fed infants (breast milk contains little vitamin D especially in vitamin D deficient mothers) of dark skinned (Asian and Afro-Caribbean) mothers and is commoner in infants of mothers who for cultural reasons cover a large part of their skin and who are on a diet with little vitamin D in it.

3. Hypocalcaemic fits or tetany should be treated with iv calcium.

General points

1. Failing to act on abnormal results is negligent. It can lead to a patient's deterioration and to a delay in treatment.

2. It is recommended that vitamin D supplementation is provided to pregnant and lactating mothers and to breast-fed and partially breast-fed infants. However, the implementation of this policy needs to be improved.

Further reading and references

Greer FR, Finberg L (2010) Rickets. http://emedicine.medscape.com/article/985510-overview

Salama MM, El-Sakka AS (2010) Hypocalcaemic seizures in breast fed infants with rickets secondary to severe maternal vitamin D deficiency. *Pak. J. Biol. Sci.* 13: 437–42. http://scialert.net/fulltext/?doi=pjbs.2010.437.442&org=11

Case 36 A febrile boy with a scald

Calum, an 18-month-old boy, attends ED with an accidental scald to his left lower leg and foot, after kicking over a cup of tea that had been left on the floor. The wound is assessed to be less than 1%, partial thickness and noncircumferential. There are no safeguarding concerns. The wound is dressed and Calum is discharged home.

Three days later Calum is brought back to the ED as he has developed vomiting and diarrhoea. At triage he is noted to have a temperature of 38.5°C, and a heart rate of 165/min. His other observations are within normal limits including a CRT of < 2 seconds, although he does not have his BP measured. He is given a dose of paracetamol and is started on an oral fluid challenge at triage.

Calum is assessed by the ED FY2 doctor, Dr Evans, 2 hours after his arrival. He is now afebrile with a heart rate of 140/min and his other observations remain within normal limits. He has tolerated his oral fluid with no further vomiting. He is found to have a macular-papular rash, with no petechiae. The burn dressing is not removed as Calum is due to be seen by the community nurses that afternoon.

Dr Evans makes a diagnosis of viral gastroenteritis. As Calum, has tolerated his fluid challenge and the fever has settled, Dr Evans plans to discharge the patient home. He discusses this with the ED registrar, Dr Riley, although Dr Evans makes no mention of Calum's recent burn. Dr Riley , agrees with Dr Evans' plan, and Calum is discharged with gastroenteritis advice.

Do you think this is an appropriate diagnosis/management plan?

That afternoon, the ED receives a blue call from an ambulance, alerting the ED that they are en route with Calum, who has a fluctuating level of consciousness. A paediatric cardiac arrest call is placed and the arrest team are present when Calum arrives.

On arrival, Calum has a temperature of 39.5°C, a heart rate of 200/min with a CRT of 2 seconds peripherally, a respiratory rate of 35/min and SaO_2 of 98% in 10L/min of O_2. The GCS is 12–13 and the nurse is unable to obtain a BP measurement. His rash has progressed to involve the whole body. Calum's burn is now undressed and shows a thick yellow crusting exudate.

The paediatric registrar, Dr Adwani, obtains peripheral iv access and sends base line bloods including blood cultures. A venous gas and FBC, are checked by near-patient testing in the ED. A diagnosis of sepsis is made and Calum is started on iv co-amoxiclav. Although he is tachycardic, Dr. Adwani is reassured by the normal CRT and prescribes maintenance iv fluids.

Is this a reasonable course of management?

The blood gas shows a partially compensated metabolic acidosis with a pH of 7.02 (normal 7.35–7.45), a pCO_2 of 3.5 kPa (4.0–6.5 kPa) a BE of −11 mmol/L (−2.5 to +2.5 mmol/L) and a lactate of 6.4 mmol/L (<2 mmol/L). The FBC shows an Hb of 12 g/dL (11–14 g/dL), a WCC of 2.3 × 10^9/L (4–11 × 10^9/L) and platelets of 80 × 10^9/L (150–400 × 10^9/L).

Dr Adwani telephones the on-call consultant, who advises that the child is likely to have toxic shock syndrome (TSS), with warm shock and asks Dr Adwani to aggressively fluid resuscitate Calum. Dr Adwani gives 2 × 20 ml/kg boluses of 0.9% Saline, but this has no effect on Calum's clinical condition.

At this stage the consultant arrives and confirms the clinical diagnosis of TSS. A further 20 ml/kg fluid bolus is given, while at the same time the local PICU and retrieval team are contacted. On their advice noradrenaline and dopamine infusions are started.

Calum is transferred to a PICU where he shows evidence of multi-organ system failure. Despite all

Avoiding Errors in Paediatrics, First Edition. Joseph E. Raine, Kate Williams and Jonathan Bonser.
© 2013 John Wiley & Sons, Ltd. Published 2013 by Blackwell Publishing Ltd.

possible therapies, he dies 24 hours later after developing the Adult Respiratory Distress Syndrome (ARDS) and becoming impossible to ventilate. The causative organism is confirmed as an exotoxin-producing strain of *Staphlococcus aureus*.

The hospital declares a serious incident and a full root cause analysis of Calum's death is undertaken.

Expert opinion

Toxic Shock Syndrome is a form of distributive shock caused by toxins produced by *Staphylococcus aureus* or *Group A Streptococcus [GAS]*. In both cases the toxin acts as a super-antigen causing a polyclonal T cell activation and then a cytokine storm, which results in multisystem organ failure.

Although associated with tampon use, 50% of cases are caused by other types of infection, commonly skin and soft tissue infections, particularly of burns or surgical wounds. *GAS* infection is also associated with recent *Varicella* infection.

The clinical diagnosis is based on a combination of fever, rash, hypotension and evidence of organ failure in 3 or more systems. As the exotoxins cause erythroderma, the capillary refill time is an unreliable sign and it is the tachycardia and hypotension that indicate the warm shock.

Once recognized the treatment is initially aggressive fluid resuscitation, then inotropic support and support of other organ systems as needed plus combination antibiotic therapy. Most patients will need to be treated in a PICU. *Staphylococcal* TSS has a mortality of 3.3% while *GAS* TSS mortality is >30%.

In this case the failure of the FY2, Dr Evans, to fully examine Calum's wound, which would have probably prompted the consideration of a wound infection, is significant and may well have contributed to Calum's death.

This was compounded by Dr Evans's failure to communicate all the relevant details of the child's case to the registrar, Dr Riley, with whom he discussed the case. Even though Dr Evans may not have been aware of the possibility of TSS, the mention to Dr Riley of a recent burn may have prompted the re-evaluation of Calum prior to discharge.

Legal comment

The family have not yet made a complaint. But if they instruct an expert to look at the case, he may well criticize the failure of Dr Evans to examine the scald wound and his failure to mention it to the registrar, Dr Riley, when Calum first returned to the hospital. But in terms of a claim in negligence, the real question is whether an examination at that time would have altered the outcome. If the correct diagnosis had been made and appropriate treatment had been administered, would Calum's life have been saved? As ever, the expert will have to provide an answer on the balance of probabilities. It appears that prompt action may well have made a difference. If so, the family will receive compensation.

Key learning points

Specific to the case

1. The presence of a fever in a child with a recent burn or other skin/soft tissue wound should always prompt consideration of a wound infection.

2. If there is a widespread rash, then the diagnosis of TSS should be considered and the child examined and, if needed, investigated for signs of sepsis and multi-organ failure.

General points

1. When junior doctors are discussing patients with senior colleagues, they should always discuss any other recent illnesses or injuries, even if they are not apparently relevant.

2. Paediatric doctors should be aware that although capillary refill time is a useful clinical sign in some forms of shock, it can be misleading in warm distributive shock.

References and further reading

Tolan RW *et al.* (2011) Pediatric Toxic Shock Syndrome. www.emedicine.medscape.com/article/969239-overview#aw2aab6b2

Venkataraman R *et al.* (2010) Toxic Shock Syndrome. www.emedicine.medscape.com/article/169177-overview

Investigating and dealing with errors

1 Introduction

Part 1 of this book looked at how errors occur. Part 2 examined detailed examples of errors. This third part looks at the mechanisms in place to pick up and then respond to errors. Those mechanisms are operated by the organization providing the healthcare (i.e. the hospital), by the professional regulatory system (NCAS, the GMC), and by the wider legal system (the Coroner, the civil or criminal Courts).

A doctor who makes an error may find himself the subject of investigations by each of these bodies. For example the doctors in the vincristine case referred to in Part 1 will have no doubt faced internal hospital investigations with a view to disciplinary proceedings.

There was certainly a police investigation and it led to a criminal trial. The death of the patient was reported to the Coroner and an Inquest was opened. The family of the patient may well have sued the hospital for damages for its negligence. The case will also certainly have come to the attention of the GMC.

Rightly or wrongly, the fact is that all these investigations will have primarily focused on how those individual doctors were to blame for what happened, and only secondarily on the defects in the system which may have contributed to the outcome.

This final part of the book gives a factual account of how these mechanisms work. We also give some practical advice. However, a doctor facing an investigation of any significance will need considerable legal and moral support, as we explain below.

2 How hospitals try to prevent errors and their recurrence

The following are the main mechanisms for picking up errors. They are themselves subject to continuous review and discussion.

Incident reporting

All NHS Trusts have systems to identify and manage risk. Staff have a duty to report not just errors but any untoward events. They must be familiar

Avoiding Errors in Paediatrics, First Edition. Joseph E. Raine, Kate Williams and Jonathan Bonser.
© 2013 John Wiley & Sons, Ltd. Published 2013 by Blackwell Publishing Ltd.

with the procedure to do so. An 'untoward event' is defined more widely than an error. It is, 'Any unintended or unexpected incident which could have or did lead to harm for one or more patients receiving NHS funded healthcare.'

This definition covers 'near misses' as well as incidents which actually caused harm. Hospital policies will give examples (or a 'trigger list') to help staff identify an 'untoward event'. Nonclinical incidents would include slips, trips and falls, violence and aggression. Clinical incidents encompass medication errors, hospital acquired infections, delays in treatment, consent issues, and the sudden death of a child. It is estimated that 10% of NHS in patients experience an adverse incident.

While there will be minor variations between different Trusts in how these reports are managed, the process would normally include these steps:
1. The staff member should verbally report the incident to the supervisor/line manager/ward manager or hospital bleep holder on duty at the time.
2. The staff member should then complete the Trust's incident report form; this form is normally located on the Trust's intranet. Most Trusts will require this form to be completed no more than 4 hours after an incident has occurred. NHS hospitals are increasingly using online forms and the most commonly used system is the Datix Software System, which in theory should make incident reporting quicker, easier and more accessible.
3. There will then be some form of internal management review; this normally has to be completed within 72 hours and includes the collation of witness statements (See Part 3, Section 8, **The role of the doctor**, for more details).
4. The incident will then be graded and, depending on the classification, further investigation may take place. If the incident is serious, a Root Cause Analysis (RCA) investigation, or an external inquiry, will need to take place (See Part 3, Section 5, **Hospital investigations**, for more details).
5. Once the appropriate level/type of investigation has taken place, an action plan will be agreed to ensure that appropriate preventative action has taken place.
6. All the staff involved in the incident will be given feedback once the investigation has been concluded. The feedback should be at departmental meetings.
7. The action plan will then be monitored.

Incident reports are transferred electronically to the National Reporting and Learning Service (NRLS) so as to create a national database. This allows trends to become apparent which may not be obvious at a local level.

Some incidents must also be reported to external bodies. The hospital policy should specify when this should happen, but examples are:
1. Untimely, unexpected and suspicious deaths should be reported to the Coroner and/or Police.
2. 'Never Events' should be reported to the NRLS. A 'Never Event' is a serious, largely preventable patient safety incident which should not occur

if appropriate preventative measures had been implemented. An example is wrong site surgery.

3. An incident that could impact on liability/indemnity cover arrangements should be reported to the NHS Litigation Authority.
4. Incidents that could involve the safeguarding of both adults or children should be reported to the local Safeguarding teams.
5. Any fatal injury in an accident connected with Trust business should be reported to the Health and Safety Executive.

A shortcoming of reporting systems is that staff may be reluctant to complete forms, partly because they are time-consuming, and partly because of concern that they will be blamed for the incident or be seen to have blamed other people. It is thought that there is significant under reporting of harmful events for these reasons, which is clearly bad practice. Furthermore, in some hospitals the investigation of errors and the provision of feedback to prevent a recurrence is poorly handled.

Whistleblowing

As well as having a policy requiring staff to report untoward incidents, all NHS Trusts should have a whistleblowing policy. This policy will protect an employee who wishes to raise a concern of general interest about the operation of the Trust. It should tell the employee whom to approach to report his concern. The relevant manager must take the disclosure seriously and must investigate it as soon as possible. Timescales will be laid down for responses. If appropriate, the issues can be fed into the incident investigation policy. A whistleblower with a genuine concern will be protected from any kind of retribution or unfavourable treatment as a result of his disclosure, provided that he acts in good faith. If he raises a concern out of malice or when he knows the facts to be untrue, then he cannot expect to be protected.

Whistleblowing policies are based on the protection afforded by the Public Interest Disclosure Act 1998. The point of the Act (which should be reflected in any policy) is to encourage disclosures, so long as they are made to the appropriate person. A person who wants to blow the whistle in public (e.g. by going to the media or to the Care Quality Commission) will not be protected unless he has attempted to get his concern investigated internally, but been ignored, or unless there is good reason to believe he would suffer if he raised it internally. Even then, it has to be an exceptionally serious matter for the protection of the Act to apply.

In January 2012 the GMC published new guidance for doctors about whistleblowing called 'Raising and Acting on Concerns about Patient Safety'. It is significant in that it places a positive professional duty on a doctor to raise concerns when he believes that patient safety is being compromised. In addition, it stipulates that a doctor *must* not enter into agreements with employers which restrict him from raising concerns about patient safety.

A doctor who finds himself under pressure to sign such an agreement must point out his professional duty not to do so.

Any member of staff can get independent advice about whistleblowing from charities such as Public Concern at Work or from trade union representatives.

Guidelines and protocols

Guidelines are systematically developed statements designed to help doctors make the right healthcare decisions. They should be statements of best practice based on a review of the current medical evidence. They should summarize the key information on a topic and should be reviewed at agreed intervals to ensure that they remain up to date and take into account new developments. Guidelines may be national, for example from NICE, or they may be issued by local organizations and adapted to suit local conditions, populations and facilities. They provide a general framework for treating patients with the aim of reducing variations in practice. A doctor can treat them as a useful source of reference, but ultimately he is not required to adhere strictly to them.

The term 'protocol' suggests a more rigid set of statements allowing little or no flexibility or variation. They provide the doctor with a precise sequence of activities to follow in the management of a specific condition. However, in practice, the terms 'guidelines' and 'protocols' are often used interchangeably.

Guidelines and protocols may need to be adjusted to meet individual circumstances. A doctor should always use his clinical judgment. However, any reasons for deviating from a guideline or protocol should be discussed with a senior doctor and carefully recorded in the patient's notes.

Guidelines and protocols can help a doctor make fewer mistakes. They can be particularly useful when a doctor faces a stressful situation. He does not need to rely solely on his memory. Online versions avoid problems of paper copies being lost and are easier to update. They can be particularly helpful for trainees, and for doctors facing an unusual situation. A review of an adverse incident can highlight the need to create a new guideline for a particular condition in order to prevent an error recurring.

Audit

Audit is the process of comparing current practice with gold standards for best practice (these can be local, national or international). The audit cycle is a process of collecting data, comparing it with gold standards and then identifying any deficiencies in practice or areas for improvement. Changes should then be implemented and the audit repeated. It should be a continuous process to ensure that standards are continuously monitored with the overall aim of improving the quality of care.

All hospitals should have audit programmes with regular audit meetings. Protocols and guidelines often provide standards for audit.

The role of audit is to promote best practice, but in so doing areas of error may be identified. It is a key component of clinical governance and hence is a tool for minimizing harm as well as maximizing quality.

Paediatric Trigger Tools

The Paediatric Trigger Tool[1] is a recent development which measures the rate of harm in healthcare by structured case note reviews. The UK tool was developed by the NHS Institution for Innovation and Improvement and was launched in 2009. It was supported by evidence from adult practice and research in Canada.

A 20-minute systematic review of case notes is performed, looking to identify key 'trigger' events which serve as clues that harm may have occurred. The notes are then further examined to see if these events did indeed result in harm. If harm occurred, it is categorized according to severity. Data can be entered on a structured record chart and uploaded via a web portal which allows the analysis of data and calculations of adverse event rates.

The aim is to identify priorities for patient safety improvements. Twenty sets of notes should be reviewed monthly, to allow improvements to be tracked over time.

The process is based on the idea that traditional voluntary incident reporting does not reliably occur and is estimated to identify only 5–10% of harmful events, whereas trigger tools detect harm rates in excess of 30%.

The emphasis is on exploring systems rather than individuals. It is not used to identify details of specific events – other tools may be needed for this. The data is intended to help minimize harm within an organization and not for comparisons between hospitals.

Appraisals

All consultants and career grade doctors are required to undergo an annual appraisal. For trainees, there is a separate system organized by the Deanery, which has many similarities. The appraisal should be private and confidential. It is based on the GMC's booklet 'Good Medical Practice' which describes the principles of good medical practice, and the standards of competence and conduct required of doctors in their professional work. The appraisal forces doctors to think about their achievements and failings in the previous year and to consider what they would like to accomplish in the forthcoming year. As well as dealing with issues such as the doctor's clinical performance and effectiveness over the previous year, the appraisal also looks at complaints (which should be reflected on and learnt from), disciplinary matters, probity, health, continuing medical education and audit. The Clinical Director or clinical lead for the department usually acts as the appraiser and ideally will have been trained in the process. Once completed, the appraiser and appraisee sign the form and send it to the hospital's Medical Director (in some institutions it may be sent to the Chief Executive) so that they are aware of any relevant issues, for example additional clinical training or disciplinary issues, which may require further action.

More recently 360 degree appraisals have also been introduced in some hospitals. This kind of appraisal requires anonymous feedback on a doctor's performance from 10–15 colleagues (doctors, nurses, secretaries). Anonymous feedback is also obtained from 20–30 patients using set forms. Many consultants find it a useful means of assessing their performance. At present it complements the standard appraisal process, but in time it may become incorporated into the standard appraisal process.

An annual appraisal will also be required as part of a doctor's GMC revalidation process (See Part 3, Section 7 (External inquiries), The GMC in future, (a) revalidation).

3   The role of hospital staff

A significant part of hospital administration is involved in risk management and in looking at the consequences of errors. The main roles/departments are as follows:

Medical Director

By law every NHS Trust has a Medical Director. He or she is a senior doctor who is responsible for patients' treatments and for making sure that medical regulations are observed and standards are met, for example: making sure patient confidentiality is protected and that medical equipment is checked and monitored.

The Medical Director is also responsible for doctors working for the Trust: for their work contracts, for supporting them in training to become specialists, especially if they get into difficulties. The Medical Director is also likely to be appointed as the GMC's Responsible Officer for revalidation (See Part 3, Section 7 (External inquiries), The GMC in future, (a) revalidation).

Clinical Director

The primary obligation of a Clinical Director, regardless of the type of facility he or she is heading, is supervision. The Clinical Director is expected to chair and coordinate employee work-related activities such as meetings and workshops. Other managerial duties include the prevention and analysis of problems before and as they occur. They must make certain that all facilities, policies and regulations are upheld and fulfilled. Lastly, a Clinical Director regularly trains and evaluates staff members.

Occupational Health Department

The Occupational Health department's purpose is to promote the physical, mental and social well-being of all staff in the organization. It tries to reduce absence because of health problems caused by working conditions. It helps to protect workers from the risks they take in their employment. In short, its aim is 'the adaption of work to man and of each man to his job' (ILO and WHO definition). The Occupational Health doctor may have a particular role in investigating clinical errors where they are thought to stem from a doctor's health problems.

The Patient Advice and Liaison Service

The Patient Advice and Liaison Service, known as PALS, aims to ensure that the NHS listens to patients, their relatives, carers and friends, answers their questions and resolves their concerns as quickly as possible.

In particular, PALS will:

- provide information about the NHS and help with any other health-related enquiry;
- help resolve concerns or problems;
- provide information about the NHS complaints procedure and how to get independent help;
- improve the NHS by listening to patient concerns, suggestions and experiences and by informing the people who design and manage services of the issues that have been raised;
- provide an early warning system for NHS Trusts and monitoring bodies by identifying problems or gaps in services and reporting them. More information can be found at the PALS website: http://www.pals.nhs.uk/.

Hospital's Legal Department

Most Trusts will have a Legal Services Department to provide a comprehensive legal service to the Trust and its employees on any matter relating to Trust business.

The main areas of responsibility are litigation (clinical and nonclinical), employment law, contract law, corporate law and document disclosure. The legal team usually manages cases referred to the Coroner and also other cases in which the Court service or police are involved. In addition, the legal team is usually available during working hours to provide advice on any legal issue which relates to the Trust's business. The most common day to day requests concern consent, parental responsibility, child protection, and compliance with Court orders.

Public Relations (PR) Department

The job of the PR and Communications departments is to raise the profile of the Trust, maintain its public and internal websites, manage press enquiries and publicize major events and projects within the Trust. It also produces the annual report and other corporate documents, as well as staff newsletters.

This department will also be involved in managing any media interest after an incident. Calls from local media should be directed to them.

Risk management

Risk management departments are responsible for the whole spectrum of things that can go wrong. This includes slips and trips involving staff, patients and the public, administrative errors that impact on patient care and clinical incidents that affect the outcome of patient care. This department also manages the business risks associated with running a NHS Board or hospital, including financial, ethical and information technology risks.

Clinical governance

Clinical governance has been defined as 'a system through which NHS organizations are accountable for continuously improving the quality of their services and safeguarding high standards of care by creating an environment in which excellence in clinical care will flourish'.[2]

It is usually the clinical governance team in a hospital which ensures that all executive directors, commissioners and other appropriate authorities and stakeholders are informed of an incident. This may include the Care Quality Commission, Monitor, the Health and Safety Executive, National Reporting and Learning Service, the NHS Litigation Authority and the police.

4   External investigators

There are external agencies whose function is to oversee the clinical risk management processes of each healthcare organization. These are the main ones:

The NHS Commissioning Board

At the time of writing, the NHS is in the process of a major new reorganization, whereby the National Patient Safety Agency (NPSA) is abolished and the NHS *Commissioning Board* is established. Its overriding role is to ensure that the NHS delivers better outcomes for patients. It works with clinical commissioning groups and the wider system to use the commissioning budget of around £80 billion a year to secure the best possible health outcomes for patients and communities. It supports quality improvement by promoting consistent national quality standards.

The National Reporting and Learning Service, previously a division of NPSA, will continue to exist, but will be managed in future by the NHS Commissioning Board. The function of this organization is to identify and reduce risks to patients receiving NHS care.

The NRLS receives local patient safety incident reports into its database. Then clinicians and safety experts analyse those reports to identify common risks and opportunities to improve patient safety. Healthcare organizations are then provided with feedback and guidance to improve patient safety.

The *National Research Ethics Service* was previously a division of the NPSA but in future will be part of the Human Research Authority.

National Clinical Assessment Service (NCAS)

NCAS was established in 2001. Its purpose is to advise healthcare organizations (both NHS and private) which are concerned about the practice of doctors, dentists or pharmacists for whom they are responsible. Its aim is to help those organizations look quickly and fairly into questions about the performance or conduct of a doctor or other healthcare professional.

A person with authority at the hospital (often, but not always the Medical Director) can telephone a NCAS adviser who will then talk through a case and advise on how to investigate further, whether to consider excluding a doctor and/or whether to implement disciplinary procedures. Advice given on the telephone will usually then be confirmed in writing. (Copies of correspondence will, in principle, be disclosable to the doctor under the Data Protection Act.) As the case develops, the NCAS adviser will continue to advise as required by the hospital. NCAS reports that over the ten years of its existence, requests for help have increased 10-fold from about 100 in its first year, to more than 1000 in 2010.

In addition to advising, NCAS will, upon request, provide clinical assessment services. An assessment of a doctor's competence cannot be carried out without his agreement. (The idea will be presented to him as the alternative to something worse, e.g. disciplinary proceedings or a GMC referral.) An assessment might be directed towards clinical concerns, health concerns, 'communicative competence' and/or behaviour concerns. NCAS reports that about one referral in 20 will involve a clinical assessment. Its published statistics show that the medical specialty most likely to be assessed is general medical practice, and that older practitioners are more likely to be assessed than younger ones. The good news is that since 2002, only 5% of NCAS assessments have concerned paediatricians.

The clinical assessment process is wide ranging and includes an occupational health assessment, a behavioural assessment, and a clinical assessment visit. There will be assessment workbook exercises and feedback from patients and peers.

The assessment will conclude with a report setting out the findings based on triangulated evidence (i.e. evidence from three different sources) and recommending the next step for both the doctor and the referrer. This will usually be a structured action plan, involving the monitoring of the doctor's performance with clearly identifiable points at which the situation is to be reviewed.

Last year (2010/2011) three out of every four practitioners assessed were continuing to do clinical work, albeit nearly half of them with some kind of restriction on their practice.

The most common clinical issues that NCAS deals with are child protection issues, and prescribing and diagnostic skills. The most common behavioural problem is communication with colleagues.

In some cases of serious concern, NCAS may advise on whether to refer to the GMC. There may even be discussions with the GMC.

From the doctor's point of view, the drawback to NCAS is that its advice is based only on what it is told by the referring organization. NCAS does not conduct its own investigation into matters save when a clinical assessment is requested. Furthermore, once its advice has been given, a Medical Director is highly likely to feel professionally obliged to follow it. Yet, because it is only advice, a doctor has no legal recourse against NCAS.

It is planned that NCAS will become 'self-funded' over the next few years. It seems that its customers (healthcare organizations) may have to pay for advice in the future. An aggrieved practitioner might feel, on the basis of the principle that he who pays the piper calls the tune, that NCAS may then become even less impartial.

The Healthcare Quality Improvement Partnership (HQIP)

The Healthcare Quality Improvement Partnership (HQIP) was established in April 2008 to promote quality in healthcare, and in particular to increase the impact that clinical audit has on healthcare quality in England and Wales. It promotes the national clinical audit programme and, with the data collected, it produces programmes for quality improvement.

The Care Quality Commission

This body was established in 2009. Its purpose is to ensure that various health services and adult social care services are meeting required standards. It does this through registration procedures and through inspections, which can be unannounced. It covers diverse services including hospitals, dentists, ambulances, care homes, family planning and slimming clinics. From 2012 its aegis extends to primary medical services and it is planned that from 2013 GPs will also be required to register.

5 Hospital investigations

Complaints management

A complaint is defined as 'an oral or written expression of dissatisfaction from an individual(s), which requires a response'.[3]

Every NHS organization must have a formal written complaints procedure. The NHS Constitution sets out the various rights of the NHS patient. In particular all patients have the right to:

- have their complaint dealt with properly and efficiently investigated;
- know the outcome of any investigation into their complaint;
- take their complaint to the Health Service Ombudsman if they are not satisfied with the way the NHS has dealt with it;
- make a claim for judicial review if they have been on the receiving end of an unlawful act or decision by an NHS body;
- to receive compensation if they have been harmed.

All NHS Trusts have, by virtue of the Health Act 2009, a duty to have regard to the NHS Constitution. The NHS Complaints Procedure requires:

1. all complaints to be registered and allocated a reference number; this will be done by the Complaints Department;
2. an acknowledgement to be sent within 3 working days;
3. all staff involved in the alleged incident to be asked to comment;
4. the Complaints Department to agree a response time with the Complainant;
5. in appropriate cases, a meeting is to be arranged with the Complainant.

A complaints investigation must comply with the following statutory requirements:

'14. *Investigation and response*

(1) *A responsible body to which a complaint is made must –*
   (a) *investigate the complaint in a manner appropriate to resolve it speedily and efficiently; and*
   (b) *during the investigation, keep the Complainant informed, as far as reasonably practicable, as to the progress of the investigation.*
(2) *As soon as reasonably practicable after completing the investigation, the responsible body must send the Complainant in writing a response, signed by the responsible person, which includes –*
   (a) *report which includes the following matters –*
      (i) *an explanation of how the complaint has been considered; and*
      (ii) *the conclusions reached in relation to the complaint, including any matters for which the complaint specifies, or the responsible body considers, that remedial action is needed; and*
   (b) *confirmation as to whether the responsible body is satisfied that any action needed in consequence of the complaint has been taken or is proposed to be taken.*'[4]

Root Cause Analysis (RCA)

The purpose of RCA is to objectively determine the underlying, as well as the obvious causes of patient incidents, thereby enabling staff and management to learn from and avoid similar incidents in the future. Its essence is to go deeper than apparent causes of events, and in particular to look at the influence of human factors.

The steps of a RCA investigation are as follows:
1. information collection;
2. information organization, including the production of a simple and tabular timeline;
3. information analysis, including identifying care and service delivery problems, contributory factors, failed and missing systems and the production of recommendations.

Serious incidents must be investigated using Root Cause Analysis. However the method can also be used for investigating all complaints. A serious incident is defined one occurring in NHS funded services and resulting in one of the following:

- unexpected or avoidable death of one or more patients, staff, visitors or members of the public;
- serious harm to one or more patients, staff, visitors or members of the public; this includes cases where life-saving or major surgical/medical intervention is required, where the incident causes permanent harm, shortens life expectancy or results in prolonged pain or psychological harm;
- a scenario which prevents or threatens to prevent a hospital's ability to continue to deliver healthcare services; for example, actual or potential loss of personal/organizational information, damage to property, reputation or the environment, or information technology failure;
- allegations of abuse;
- adverse media coverage or public concern about the organization or the wider NHS;
- one of the core set of 'Never Events' as updated on an annual basis and currently including:
  - wrong site surgery
  - retained instrument postoperation
  - wrong route for administration of chemotherapy
  - misplaced naso-gastric or oro gastric tube, not detected prior to use
  - intravenous administration of wrongly selected concentrated potassium chloride.

Ideally RCA investigations should not be undertaken by a single investigator, but by a team. NHS Trusts should provide training to those who are expected to undertake an RCA investigation.

Apologies

A complaint against a doctor may be resolved, or it may lead to one or more further, more demanding investigations.

Patients often say that if they had received a sincere apology from the doctor for the error, they would not have pursued a claim or other form of complaint. Indeed, the received wisdom is that an apology often does satisfy a patient and/or the family and may resolve the problem. However, this is not always the case. Often a doctor may quite justifiably believe that he should not be blamed for a poor outcome. Lawyers too prefer claims to be investigated before any shortcomings in the standard of care are admitted. If an apology which admits fault has already been made, then this could prejudice the case, making it difficult to defend what may in fact be an eminently defensible case.

Sometimes the answer to the question whether a doctor should apologize or not will be obvious. Where there has been an obvious mistake in a medication dosage, for example, a prompt apology may well be advisable.

The NHS Litigation Authority in 2009 published a letter to all NHS bodies, encouraging meaningful apologies to patients and their relatives. The letter was endorsed by each of the MDOs, who said that 'Any patient who has had the misfortune to suffer through an error of whatever nature should receive a full explanation and a genuine apology. We encourage members to adopt this approach. There are no legal concerns about taking this course of action: it is quite different from admitting liability.'

The best advice to a doctor who is in doubt is to discuss the matter with his colleagues, his MDO and/or the Trust's complaints manager.

Disciplinary procedures

A possible consequence of committing an error (or, perhaps more likely, a series of errors) is an investigation under the hospital's disciplinary procedure, and in particular under the procedure for dealing with issues of capability.

A doctor's contract of employment with his NHS Trust will incorporate within it the Trust's disciplinary procedure for medical staff. Since 2005 every NHS Trust in England has been required to model its disciplinary procedure for doctors on the framework published by the Department of Health in 2003 called 'Maintaining High Professional Standards in the Modern NHS' (known as 'MHPS'). This framework was intended to cure the defects of the previous slow and cumbersome process, which involved a legal chairman and lawyers acting for each side. In particular, the old system often led to prolonged suspensions of doctors for months, sometimes even years.

The new procedure requires every Trust to involve NCAS at an early stage. The intention is to reduce the need to use disciplinary procedures at all. However, in some circumstances, NCAS will advise a Trust that a case should be treated as a disciplinary matter.

MHPS divides all disciplinary matters into two groups, those involving issues of capability and those of misconduct. Capability issues arise, according to MHPS, when an employer considers that there has been a clear failure by an individual to deliver an adequate standard of care or standard of management, whether through lack of knowledge, ability or consistently poor performance. Underlying these problems there may be a lack of team working skills, practice which is out of date or just plain incompetence.

Misconduct, on the other hand, is a category concerned with inappropriate behaviour. Where the misconduct has nothing to do with the practice of medicine, the doctor will go through the same disciplinary procedure as any other employee of the Trust. If, however, the alleged misconduct is associated with the practice of medicine (for example, if it is said that the doctor lied to cover up medical mistakes, was unnecessarily rude to patients or colleagues, or had an inappropriate relationship with a patient), then it is a question of professional misconduct, and the special procedures for medical staff laid down in MHPS will apply.

MHPS goes on to say that any concerns about capability or conduct relating to a doctor in a recognized training grade should be considered initially as a training issue and dealt with via the educational supervisor and college or clinical tutor. A disciplinary hearing for a doctor in training is therefore comparatively rare, especially a hearing about his capability.

An outline of the disciplinary procedure applicable in both capability and conduct matters is as follows:

1. A Case Manager is appointed at the Trust who must decide initially whether the case needs to be dealt with formally or informally. The Case Manager must have had no involvement in the issues under investigation. Often the Clinical Director will take this role.

2. If the Case Manager wants to look at the case informally, then with the assistance of NCAS, solutions involving training and support may be considered. These are often sufficient measures, particularly to deal with capability cases.

3. If the case is thought to require formal action, then the Case Manager should appoint a Case Investigator. The Case Investigator is likely to be another doctor at the Trust, probably from a different discipline. Again, he should have had no previous involvement in the issues in the case.

4. In the meantime, the Case Manager must also consider whether the duty to protect patients means that the doctor in question should be excluded from work or his clinical duties should be restricted during the investigation. The Case Manager may also consider whether a referral to the GMC is required, even at this early stage.

5. A further measure which can be considered in serious cases is the issue of an 'alert letter' warning other Trusts and private employers that the doctor is under investigation.

6. The Case Investigator then conducts an investigation, usually by interviewing relevant staff members and/or patients. Sometimes an expert report is commissioned.

7. The doctor should be informed of the investigation, and the specific allegations or concerns which are under consideration. He should be copied into all the paperwork and given an opportunity to put his point of view to the investigator.

8. The Case Investigator then writes a report to the Case Manager making recommendations for the future management of the case.

9. The Case Manager then decides whether or not to hold a formal disciplinary hearing.

10. If there is to be a disciplinary hearing, then whether the issues are ones of capability or professional misconduct or a mixture of the two, the disciplinary panel must consist of three people, one of whom must be a medically qualified person not employed by the Trust (but appointed by the Trust). (The other two members will be from within the Trust.)

Most Trusts' disciplinary procedures provide that a doctor may be represented before a disciplinary panel by a colleague or friend, but not by a lawyer. However, in view of the very serious consequences to a doctor of a dismissal by his Trust (it can make it potentially difficult for him to practise his profession at all, since the NHS holds a near monopoly on the practice of medicine), it has been suggested in a judgment from the High Court that in certain serious cases, it may well be a breach of the doctor's human rights not to allow him legal representation. This was sufficient to persuade many Trusts to allow legal representation in cases where the doctor's job was at risk. However, the argument was recently considered by the Court of Appeal and rejected. It was held that a doctor's "human right" to practise his profession was not engaged in local disciplinary proceedings, so that his rights are limited to a hearing which is conducted in accordance with MHPS (which does not provide for legal representation).

The outcome of a disciplinary hearing will be recorded in a letter to the doctor. The Panel must say which allegations have been found proved, and give a brief account of its reasons. It must then go on to consider what disciplinary sanction to apply in the light of its findings, namely whether the doctor should be dismissed from his post or given a warning (oral or written) or whether no action is necessary. In cases where the doctor is dismissed, the Trust is highly likely to then refer the doctor to the GMC for an investigation into his fitness to practise.

The rights of the dismissed doctor are to appeal under the Trust's internal appeal procedure. He can also take his case to the Employment Tribunal if he considers the dismissal has been unfair, or the result of discrimination on the grounds of race, sex or age. Proceedings in the Employment Tribunal must be issued promptly (i.e. within three months) of the dismissal.

Sometimes a disciplinary procedure can be settled by way of a Compromise Agreement between the doctor as employee and the Trust as employer. Such an agreement may be a way for the doctor to avoid the stigma of a dismissal, agree the terms of a reference and any financial package. For the Trust, it may be a way to resolve potentially messy and expensive litigation.

6 Legal advice – where to get it and how to pay

If, despite a doctor's best intentions and endeavours, he finds himself on the wrong end of a complaint or an investigation, as described in this section, he is likely to be catapulted from the more or less comfortable and familiar environment of the hospital ward into an alien, possibly hostile world, very different from his usual work experience. This is a world governed by legal rules, deadlines and procedures. The doctor will need assistance to guide him through this unfamiliar territory. Colleagues may offer advice and, for more minor complaints, this may be enough. But if the complaint is at all serious, then he will require legal advice. After all, a complaint could be the beginning of a process which will end with limits on his ability to practise, the payment of damages (which could even run to millions of pounds), and a requirement to pay the legal costs incurred by the child and his family. Then there are the legal costs incurred by the lawyers representing the individual doctor or the clinical team. The level of these costs will usually be based on the time spent on the case, but bills of tens of thousands of pounds would not be unusual for a case of moderate complexity.

Who pays these legal bills? The answer depends on a number of factors, including the nature of the initial complaint, how it develops and in what capacity the doctor provided treatment to the patient.

NHS treatment

(a) Negligence claims
All doctors employed in NHS hospitals are covered for claims against them through the hospital's indemnity scheme. This means that the payment of both damages and bills for legal advice on claims will be organized through the National Health Service Litigation Authority in England, Welsh Health Legal Services in Wales, the individual Health Boards and Trusts in Northern Ireland and the Central Legal Office in Scotland. These bodies will organize legal representation and make decisions about the conduct of the case. The paediatrician involved in the treatment of the child will be expected to cooperate with the lawyers appointed by these public health bodies to defend the interests of the hospital trust.

(b) Patient complaint
A patient complaint either to the hospital or to the Health Service Ombudsman will often be dealt with through the Trust's complaints manager, who will coordinate any legal advice that is necessary. The Trust will, therefore, be responsible for the legal bills incurred. However, in an exceptional case, a doctor may wish to get his own independent legal advice.

(c) Inquests and fatal accident inquiries
The hospital Trust will organize the provision of legal advice for its clinicians and other staff at an Inquest. However, if there are conflicts between clinicians about the treatment leading up to the child's death, then a paediatrician may prefer to be personally represented at an Inquest, so that his own actions can be defended in an appropriate fashion. He cannot usually expect his costs to be paid by the hospital in those circumstances.

(d) Criminal inquiries

Sometimes a hospital Trust may pay for some of the initial defence costs of a criminal investigation. But this will depend on the nature of the case. The Trust may, for example, fund defence costs where the criminal charges arise from an apparent system failure. But the Trust may well conclude that the allegations are personal to the treating paediatrician and should be dealt with by him. In general, criminal investigations will be personal to the clinician.

(e) General Medical Council

Complaints to the GMC will be considered personal to the paediatrician. Accordingly, legal bills and the provision of legal services will not be covered by a hospital Trust.

Medical Defence Organization

It is clear that circumstances may well arise in which a doctor needs his own legal advice. This is where the Medical Defence Organisation (MDO) comes to the doctor's aid.

Until recently there were only three indemnity organizations offering legal assistance to doctors in the United Kingdom, namely the Medical Protection Society (MPS), the Medical Defence Union (MDU), and the Medical and Dental Defence Union of Scotland (MDDUS). Now there are a number of other options, but these three organizations still look after the interests of the vast majority of UK clinicians. There are variations in the kinds of indemnity they offer, from insurance based cover to discretionary cover or a combination. The doctor looking for MDO cover must look carefully at the terms and discuss them with the MDO in order to decide what kind of cover best suits him. The MDO websites each give a brief account of what is on offer.

Whatever their differences, in essence, the MDOs offer members professional and legal advice. If a doctor is a member of one of these organizations, then subject to the terms of his cover, he can call on that organization to come to his assistance in his time of need. All the MDOs offer telephone helplines, whereby a clinician can talk to a Medico-Legal Advisor on professional matters of concern, small or large. They lend a kindly ear.

To establish which cover is most appropriate, we strongly recommend that doctors contact the MDOs to find out their terms and what they mean in theory and in practice.

So, although paediatricians are automatically covered against expenses arising out of negligence claims incurred in their NHS hospital work, they still need MDO cover for support in disciplinary proceedings and criminal investigations. The MDOs will also advise on whether there is a need for personal legal representation at an Inquest and if so, they will often provide it.

Private work

If a paediatrician undertakes private hospital work, then he will also need MDO cover against all types of claim or complaint arising from this work.

We have used the word 'need'. Is this overstating the case? There was talk in the Houses of Parliament a few years ago about whether clinicians should be legally required to have their own indemnity cover, but there was no formal debate and no legislation was drafted or passed. So it is not compulsory (although most private hospitals make it a condition of its contract with a doctor). But is it worth the risk of not having cover? If a complaint is made, then the costs and the damages could be crippling and the stress considerable. What MDO membership provides is support and a measure of peace of mind to the unfortunate clinician who is subject to a complaint or claim.

7   External inquiries

The Health Service Ombudsman

A Complainant may not be satisfied with the outcome of a complaint. In that case the hospital will tell him of his right to ask the Health Service Commissioner ('HSC', often known as the 'Health Service Ombudsman'), to investigate. This is the last port of call for a person with a complaint about NHS services.

A complainant can only approach the Ombudsman when the local complaints procedure has been concluded. The function of the Ombudsman is, upon request and at his/her discretion, to investigate an alleged injustice or hardship caused by a failure in administration or service in the NHS.

If the Ombudsman takes on the case (and he/she does not have to do so) he/she has powers to call for relevant documents to be produced. Arrangements will be made for the main protagonists to be interviewed. The interviewees will be sent copies of their interview notes. The hospital will be sent a copy of the draft report, and given the opportunity to comment on it. In practice, the report will go through several drafts before it is concluded.

The report will comment on the standard of care and service found in the particular case. The Ombudsman cannot *require* any specific steps to be taken to remedy any hardship. He/she can only make recommendations. However those recommendations do have a strong moral force, particularly given the power to 'name and shame'. Generally, apologies or explanations to the complainant and/or payment of money as compensation will be recommended. The Ombudsman may also recommend ways to improve the service found to be at fault. For example, the current Ombudsman (Anne Abrahams) has recently published a high profile report called 'Care and Compassion', reciting her findings at a number of NHS institutions following complaints about poor care for the elderly. It can be seen that, as resources in the NHS are pruned down, the Ombudsman could play an important role in setting and maintaining standards of provision.

When the role of Health Service Ombudsman was first established, questions of clinical judgement by an individual doctor were specifically excluded from his remit. This has subsequently changed, and so the Ombudsman can and does now comment on the clinical judgements made by individual doctors, especially when an issue is whether those judgements have led to injustice and hardship. The Ombudsman will usually appoint Independent Assessors from the relevant medical speciality to advise on such questions. The conclusion on such questions will be based both on the facts and on the relevant professional standards (i.e. for doctors the *Bolam Standard* as described in Part 1).

Once concluded, the report is put before Parliament. It is also available on the Internet. It is in the public domain. A doctor who is exposed to the risk of criticism in this report may be well advised to ask his MDO for support in corresponding with the Ombudsman before it is published. Otherwise, his only recourse is by way of Judicial Review in the High Court, which may possibly provide a remedy if the Ombudsman's reasoning is significantly faulty or he has exceeded his remit.

Negligence claims and the litigation process

If a family issues a claim against an NHS hospital about a doctor's treatment of their child, or against the doctor personally in respect of private treatment, then either the Trust or the doctor's MDO will instruct solicitors to investigate the claim and to defend it, if that is appropriate. The solicitors will deal with the day to day management of the case, responding to correspondence from the family's legal team and attending procedural hearings at Court. They will keep the Trust, or the MDO and the doctor himself abreast of developments. One of the roles of the solicitor acting on behalf of a clinician is to minimize the worry for him.

In practical terms, a doctor's initial involvement in a claim will be a meeting with the solicitor to discuss his treatment of the child. The solicitor will normally draft a statement summarizing that treatment and will ask the doctor to approve its contents. This will be used to obtain expert opinion on the case. The solicitor may send the doctor various documents, such as the medical records, the family's statements, the reports of the experts for the Trust and those for the family. He may ask for comments on these documents.

If the case appears defensible, then the legal team will wish to test the evidence and will arrange a conference with Counsel, that is, a meeting with a barrister. The doctor will normally be required to attend such a meeting. The barrister will question him closely on his treatment of the child and ask the experts to comment on that treatment. It may be that the legal team will need two or three conferences before a final decision is made to defend the case in Court or to reach a settlement with the family. In rough terms, it will probably take three years from the first notification of the claim until a case comes to trial. However, the vast majority of claims are settled before trial, in some cases because the Claimant withdraws or in others because the Defendant makes an offer.

Negligence claims make only a relative small call on a doctor's time. The damages and costs payable to the family should come out of government funds or from the coffers of an MDO. Such claims do not attract any sanction in themselves to affect a doctor's ability to work as a doctor.

Coroner's Court

In England, Wales and Northern Ireland where there is a sudden death of which the cause is unknown, where there has been a violent or unnatural death, or where there has been a death in custody, the case has to be referred to the Coroner for an inquest, or inquiry. (In Scotland, there is a different procedure, which we describe below.)

The Coroner's role is to answer four simple factual questions:
1. Who died?
2. When did he or she die?
3. Where did he or she die?
4. How did he or she die?

In practice, it is the latter question which tends to occupy the coroner's time. When he explores this question, it is important to understand that, in principle, he is not allowed to ask questions which tend to ascribe blame or responsibility. He should restrict himself to the bare facts. In practice, however, the question of how someone died often tends to raise just such questions.

The Coroner will gather evidence from most of those involved. His enquiries will be assisted by the expert opinion of the pathologist who carries out the postmortem examination. He may also seek other expert opinion, medical or nonmedical, to help him reach a conclusion.

If you are asked to assist a Coroner's enquiry, you will be asked to provide a report outlining your involvement. As this will be read not only by the Coroner, but also possibly by the other witnesses, it may be important to seek advice about it. Your employing Trust's lawyers will usually be able to assist and advise you. Failing that, you should seek advice from your MDO.

Unless the Coroner decides, having looked at the papers, that the death was, after all, a natural one which he has no duty to investigate, he will hold a public hearing by way of investigation. Witnesses, including the doctors involved, may be called to give evidence.

The Coroner's Court is not like other courts. It is not an adversarial procedure, no one is on trial, there are no sides or parties, and no prosecution or defence. Instead, there are just persons with an interest in the proceedings. These characteristics are unique in the English legal system and of ancient origin.

The Coroner runs the Court. Thus all witnesses are called by the Coroner and he asks them most of the questions. The Coroner directs the case, which is driven by his opinion. In certain limited circumstances, such as a death in custody, a jury is required to hear the evidence and reach a verdict.

Others with an interest in the proceedings, such as the family or the hospital, also get an opportunity to ask questions of witnesses. The Coroner must ensure that only questions which are relevant to the Inquest are put to the witnesses, that is to say, relevant to the four factual matters he is required to investigate.

Sometimes the family of the deceased feels someone, or some organization (such as a hospital) is to blame for the death. They see the inquest as an opportunity to explore and expose that fault. While, in principle, the Coroner is not allowed to make findings of fault, the question 'how' someone died often does beg the question. For example, if someone dies unexpectedly, the investigation may focus on how a delay in treatment contributed to the death. In addition, the Coroner has the power to make a finding of 'neglect' in certain extreme cases of a total failure to provide basic care and attention when it was obviously required. The family may ask the Coroner to make such a finding, for example, in a case where the patient was left waiting on a trolley for treatment for an unacceptably long time.

For a doctor, it is an obvious occupational hazard that a patient might die unexpectedly. If a doctor is only asked to attend an Inquest once or twice in his career, he will have been fortunate. He is likely to feel uncomfortable anyway, but especially if he knows the case is a contentious one. Normally, the doctor's employing trust would provide any legal representation considered necessary for staff who are giving evidence. But there are unfortunate occasions when the Trust feels unable to provide representation for a particular doctor. Equally, a doctor may feel he cannot be confident his Trust will provide him with adequate legal support or he may feel he needs very particular support. In those cases, it may be appropriate for an him to have his own lawyer at the Inquest to look after his interests. The MDO will give advice on this situation, and if appropriate, will instruct a lawyer.

Having heard the evidence, the Coroner (or perhaps the jury) will deliver his 'verdict'. Traditionally, this was limited to death by natural causes, or accident or misadventure (which means an unintended consequence of an intentional act – an example would be a surgical mishap), suicide, unlawful killing or an open verdict (to name the most common). As already mentioned, the Coroner might add a rider of 'neglect' to some verdicts. This is a finding a hospital will be at pains to avoid.

However, instead of the traditional brief verdict, there is now a trend for Coroners to return a 'narrative verdict'. This is a short factual summary, usually only four or five lines long. It is meant to give a more satisfactory outcome to the hearing, which may have been an emotional trauma for the family, than the standard words.

Inquests are held in public, and there are often reports of them in the local or even national press. Furthermore, as a result of the evidence he has heard, the Coroner may announce at the conclusion of the inquest that he intends to make a report to a relevant authority with the power to take action to prevent the recurrence of a fatality similar to that just investigated. In an extreme case, he may report a doctor to the GMC and or to the police. Accordingly, it is important that the doctor prepares his evidence carefully.

Fatal Accident Inquiries

In Scotland, there is a different procedure for investigating the circumstances of a death. Under the Fatal Accident and Sudden Death Inquiry (Scotland) Act 1976, the Procurator Fiscal can investigate any death which is sudden, suspicious, unexplained or which occurred in circumstances that give rise to serious public concern. Some investigations are mandatory, namely cases of death in custody or as a result of an accident at work. In a minority of these investigations, the Procurator Fiscal will call for a hearing, called a Fatal Accident Inquiry. That hearing takes place before a Sheriff in the Sheriff Court. Acting in the public interest, the Procurator Fiscal will present the evidence. Other interested parties may be represented by lawyers (and often are). The Sheriff must determine:

(a) where and when the death took place;
(b) the cause of death;
(c) any reasonable precautions whereby the death might have been avoided;
(d) any defects in the system of working which contributed to the death;
(e) any other relevant circumstances.

Unlike the Coroner's proceedings, questions of fault are very much in issue in these proceedings, which are therefore often quite high profile.

Criminal matters

Sometimes things can go very badly wrong. A patient may make an allegation against a doctor of a crime, perhaps of fraud or perhaps of indecency. A patient may die unexpectedly shortly after receiving treatment. In these cases, the matter is passed to the police to investigate.

Initially the police will take an overview. They will have to obtain evidence to support the allegation. This might be a postmortem report, or if it is an allegation from a patient, then a statement from the patient concerned.

Then the police will want to speak to the doctor.

It cannot be sufficiently stressed how important it is for the doctor to seek advice and assistance if he knows or suspects that there is or may be a police investigation.

The police do not have 'chats', even though that is what they might call it when they contact the doctor. In fact the doctor will be interviewed under caution and that discussion will be recorded.

The police station interview will, by the very nature of it, be an alien, unfamiliar and intimidating experience. It is not at all like it is on 'The Bill'. The police now have the power to arrest whenever they feel it is necessary. The doctor's definition of 'necessary' is likely to be different from theirs. In short, if a doctor is to be interviewed, he should anticipate that he may well be arrested.

Proper preparation for any interview with the police is vital. It is often said that cases are not won at the police station stage, but they can certainly be lost if the foundation of the doctor's case is insufficiently robust.

Preparation may include requesting a second postmortem. It will certainly include lengthy meetings between the doctor and his legal and medical defence team, to analyse in depth the doctor's recollection of events. In most cases, a statement will be prepared to help the doctor and act as an aide memoire in the interview. In many cases, the doctor will be advised to simply read the statement and answer no further questions.

At the start of the interview, the doctor will be 'cautioned'. This is the form of words used to ensure the police can record anything he says in answer to their questions. The words of the caution are, 'You do not have to say anything, but it may harm your defence if you do not mention when questioned something which you later rely on in court. Anything you do say may be given in evidence.' The effect of this is that the doctor's initial account must be as comprehensive as possible. The Court could make adverse inferences about any future additions to his account, for example when he gives evidence at trial.

Thankfully, most police officers realize that doctors are busy professionals. They will try to arrange a mutually convenient time for him to attend the police station. However some officers still like the dawn raid. Even if this happens, the doctor is entitled to representation. He should try to contact his MDO, but if that fails there is always a duty solicitor available to assist.

Following the interview, there will be a period of waiting. The police will have other enquiries and when they are complete they will have to seek advice from their own lawyers at the Crown Prosecution Service (CPS). The more complex the case, the longer the waiting. In the more complex manslaughter cases the waiting can even run to a couple of years.

The prosecution has to prove, so that the jury is sure of guilt, both that the act happened and the mental element of the offence. The mental element is usually (but not always) that the accused intended to do what is alleged. However, the charge of Gross Negligence Manslaughter is slightly different. For this charge, the jury has four questions to decide:
1. Was there a duty of care?
2. Was that duty breached?
3. Did the breach cause the death? And
4. Was the negligence so 'gross' that it was criminal?

If everything goes well, the doctor will in due course be told that there is no further action. That is the end of the police investigation. However, the

Trust could still investigate and the police are also likely to pass their file to the GMC which will conduct its own investigation.

If it does not go well, the doctor will be charged. Whilst all criminal cases start in the Magistrates Court, those involving doctors are often more serious and so will be transferred to the Crown Court for trial. Any trial could be many months in the future. In the meantime, the employing trust and the GMC may each take action in the interim to restrict or suspend the doctor's ability to practise.

In any dealings with the police or Courts, remember paragraph 58 of Good Medical Practice (GMP). This states:

> 'you must inform the GMC *without delay* [emphasis added] if, anywhere in the world you have accepted a caution, *been charged with* [emphasis added] or found guilty of a criminal offence . . .'

However, and somewhat confusingly, the caution given at the beginning of an interview is different from the 'caution' one might receive as a penalty for a minor offence. The GMC requires the penalty of a caution to be reported, not the one given during a police interview. At paragraph 58 of GMP, the GMC means the penalty of a caution must be reported, *not* the one given during a police interview.

As an alternative to either a caution or a charge, the Police may issue a fixed penalty notice. Such notices can now be issued for a wide range of matters, not just speeding and parking offences. Once again, somewhat confusingly, whether or not you have to report these to the GMC depends upon whether they are 'upper' or 'lower' tier matters. We suggest doctors take advice from their MDO to help guide them.

If convicted of offences of fraud, sexual assault or manslaughter the risk of a prison sentence is high. However each case is dealt with on its own facts and thus imprisonment is not inevitable.

Thankfully, prosecutions are very rare and even when prosecuted, acquittal rates are high.

The child death review processes

These are relatively new processes, introduced to examine the circumstances of and the lessons to be learned from children's deaths across the country.

They are the result of a report written by Baroness Kennedy in 2004, which focused on sudden and unexpected deaths in infancy.

Her recommendations were then taken up in a government report called 'Working Together to Safeguard Children' in 2006. The government extended her recommendations not just to unexpected deaths, but to *all* deaths of children (i.e. under 18 years). The process has become a statutory requirement since April 2008. There are two main elements to this process which are the rapid response following the unexpected death of a child, and the Child

Death Overview Panel (CDOP) which reviews the deaths of all children up to 18 years of age.

Unexpected deaths and the rapid response

In the case of an *unexpected* death (which is defined as when death was not anticipated 24 hours beforehand, or when there was an unexpected collapse which led to death), the key professionals who had been involved with the child are required to come together in a 'rapid response' meeting to enquire into and evaluate the child's death.

These professionals might include paediatricians, GPs, health visitors, school nurses, teachers, the police, social services etc. It falls to the 'designated paediatrician' to organize the rapid response meetings and to ensure that all the relevant professionals are included and that they contribute fully to information sharing. When the death has occurred in hospital, the hospital's serious incident protocol should also be followed (see Part 3, Section 2 (How hospitals try to prevent errors and their recurrence), Incident reporting). The Coroner will also be involved, although he will not usually attend the rapid response meetings. He will, however, be informed of the information gathered through the rapid response process in the form of a written report completed by the paediatrician. Such reports are also shared with the pathologist undertaking the PM (if there is one).

In most cases of an unexpected death, but particularly when the child has died at home, a senior healthcare professional (who may well be a paediatrician) and a police officer investigating on behalf of the Coroner, should visit the home together to talk to the parents and inspect the environment in which the child died. They have to have in mind the possibility that abuse or neglect have led to or contributed to the child's death, and that there may be other children in the home who need to be protected.

The Royal College of Paediatricians recommends that this joint visit takes place within 24 hours of the death. For the police it is a priority that they visit the scene of death within the first hour to ensure that the scene is secured and that any evidence is gathered should there be criminal proceedings. The need for the police to gather evidence in this way does not preclude a later joint visit. The joint visit provides an opportunity for the paediatrician to see the home environment and the room in which the child died (noting features such as bedding, environmental temperature, furniture positioning, potential hazards, the condition of the housing and so forth) as well as an opportunity to tell the parents of the child about both the child death review processes and the Coroner's procedures, including the postmortem examination.

It is not hard to appreciate how difficult this interview is likely to be. A newly traumatized family will not be able to take in all that is going on and may be highly suspicious that the authorities are intruding on their grief. It is good practice to leave them some written material summarizing what will happen, including some useful contacts for further support for the family.

In particular, it is important that the family understand that medical or other confidential information gathered in the course of these enquiries will be shared among all the professionals involved, including the police. Normal rules on medical confidentiality are suspended in these circumstances.

The team involved in the rapid response will have a discussion shortly after the initial postmortem results are available to review all the information which has been gathered. This will ideally be within a week of the death. Consideration must be given at this case discussion to whether there are any 'safeguarding issues' which should trigger other processes.

A report is then produced for the Coroner (and the pathologist where there is a PM) which includes a review of the child's relevant medical, social and educational records. Ideally this will be within 28 days of the death. It will include certain data about the child in accordance with nationally agreed standards.

Finally, once all the information has been gathered and the final results of the PM are available (this may take 3 or more months), there will be a case discussion meeting of the members of the rapid response team. This meeting will be chaired by the 'designated paediatrician'. The purpose of this discussion is to identify the cause of death and any factors that may have contributed to it, to identify any lessons which should be learnt, and to plan future support for the family. This meeting must explicitly discuss whether abuse or neglect is thought to have contributed to the death. If there is no evidence of this, it should be expressly recorded in the minutes of the meeting.

The record of this case discussion along with copies of any other relevant information are sent to the Child Death Overview Panel.

The Child Death Overview Panel

The CDOP is the multi-agency panel responsible for reviewing all deaths of children resident in a given locality. It is constituted as a subgroup of the Local Safeguarding Children Board (LSCB). It has a fixed core membership, and invites other professionals and experts to attend meetings on an as required basis. The CDOP meets regularly, typically 2–4 monthly, depending on the number of deaths in the area.

All deaths of children, unexpected or expected must be reported by the same medical professional who confirmed the death to the Local Safeguarding Children Board (LSCB). In practice the notification needs to be sent to a 'single point of contact' (SPOC) who is integral to the workings of the CDOP. The work of the CDOP is to identify from the paper based reviews any patterns or trends in the local data and to recommend areas of improvement for service delivery. The CDOP is particularly interested in looking at whether in each case there has been effective inter-agency working to safeguard the welfare of children, whether the professionals involved have acted appropriately, and whether there are lessons to be learnt. Where there are recommendations for changes in practice, this is disseminated to all relevant services by the

CDOP and is followed up to ensure that the necessary changes have been made. The CDOP also deals with situations where there are concerns about the information or response from the service provider and with cases where there are concerns about professional practice.

The CDOP should involve families in the process by encouraging them to ask questions or to express their views about the services. This information is presented at the CDOP meeting along with all the other information and the families are given feedback about the recommendations of the panel. The other area of work for the CDOP is the the provision of bereavement support for the families.

Individual anonymized case summaries are submitted to central government to contribute to national data collection. An annual report summarizing the work of the CDOP is submitted for scrutiny to the LSCB.

Conclusion

The RCPCH has published guidance on the Child Death review processes, emphasizing the key role to be played by paediatricians both in the rapid response teams and in the Child Death Overview Panels. 'Paediatricians should be actively involved in programmes that reduce hazards to health, especially those that may result in death in the child population.'

The guidance from the RCPCH notes that the Child Death Review processes could come to be seen as an exercise in laying blame, whether on social services, hospitals or parents, and advises, 'It should be made clear to all involved that the process of investigation is focused on learning and not on blame.'[6]

Public inquiry

Public Inquiries might take place where:
- there has been a widespread loss of life;
- there are threats to public health or safety;
- there is a failure of duty by a statutory body to protect individuals.

However, there is no definitive list of events that will trigger the need for a public inquiry. A single death can lead to an enquiry, such as the child protection case of Victoria Climbié. An example of a medical inquiry is the Bristol Royal Infirmary Inquiry into paediatric heart surgery.

The Chairman of a public inquiry has the power to require witnesses to give evidence upon oath and to provide documents. Anyone refusing to comply could be charged with a criminal offence. However, the Chairman has a duty to act fairly to witnesses. Accordingly, any witness who is at risk of being criticized in the report of the Inquiry should be warned of that possibility before he gives evidence. The Chairman should send that person a letter, setting out the potential criticism and the evidence which supports it. That person should be given an opportunity to respond to the criticism.

A doctor who receives such a letter should certainly contact his MDO for assistance.

General Medical Council in practice

There are now approximately 231,000 doctors registered with the GMC and subject to its regulations. The statutory purpose of the GMC set out in the Medical Act of 1983 is to 'protect, promote and maintain the health and safety of the public by ensuring proper standards in the practice of medicine'.

Over the last seven years or so the GMC Fitness to Practise Procedures have been substantially reformed. These reforms were designed to reassure the public, in the wake of some well publicized scandals, that concerns about substandard doctors are being dealt with efficiently and promptly. The most recent reform, introduced in June 2012, is the creation of the Medical Practitioners' Tribunal Service. This body is part of the GMC, but is described as operationally separate from it. Its function is to run the various Panel hearings, so that the adjudication of cases is demonstrably separate from the investigation and prosecution of cases by the GMC.

Most complaints to the GMC are from members of the public, but a substantial minority come from a public health body or from the Police. In the case of a referral by the Police or the doctor's employing hospital, it is likely to be the result of an investigation or criminal procedures, and the doctor will probably have been told of the referral. In the case of a patient complaint, though, the doctor might well be taken by surprise when he receives a letter from the GMC.

Statistically, as a paediatrician you are unlikely to come to the GMC's attention. For example, only 5% of the 5773 complaints made to the GMC in 2009 concerned paediatricians. Not all those complaints related to clinical matters. Furthermore, roughly half of the 5% were closed with no further action taken. Only two paediatricians were actually referred to a Fitness to Practise Panel Hearing that year. Despite this, in recent years, paediatric cases at the GMC have provided some of the most attention grabbing headlines: children's heart surgery in Bristol, Dr Wakefield and the MMR vaccine, Professor Southall and child protection cases. Though few paediatricians will have the misfortune to receive a GMC letter, the effects on those who do can be profound.

This section explains what that letter from the GMC may contain, its potential consequences and what the doctor needs to do to protect himself.

Nature of the letter and the complaint

Enclosed with the letter from the GMC will be a copy of the complaint. The letter will inform the doctor that the GMC are starting to investigate the complaint.

The variety of circumstances that might lead to a GMC referral are, of course, infinite and can touch on any aspect of practice, not just clinical judgement. Often the complaint will refer to a poorly conducted medical investigation and to a bad outcome from treatment. But other common complaints concern a doctor's health (that is, that poor mental or physical health is impairing his ability to practise effectively), or dishonesty (such as false claims on a CV, failure to disclose a conviction, altering medical records), to affairs with patients or criminal investigations (fraud, sexual assault, drink driving).

The letter will invite the doctor to comment on what the complainant has to say. He should get advice from his MDO on whether to send a response. He may be anxious to put his side of the story as soon as possible, but it is not always wise to do so at this early stage.

Case investigation

The GMC has a service target of six months for concluding its investigations. So, after the initial letter, it could be some time before the doctor hears again. Enquiries will include a letter to the doctor's employers asking if there are any concerns about him. If, on completing their investigations, the case managers decide to proceed with the case, then the results of the investigation will be presented to him in a further letter, accompanied by a bundle of documents. This is known as a 'Rule 7 letter'. It sets out a series of allegations and the doctor will be asked to comment in writing before the Case Examiners decide what course of action to take. His reply to the Rule 7 letter is his major opportunity to persuade the GMC's Case Examiners that the allegations are unwarranted and that the case should be dropped at this preliminary stage.

The doctor is likely to feel very strongly about the allegations and the temptation is to express himself in emotional language. But this would be a mistake. Florid language is taken by the GMC as evidence that he lacks insight. This is the cardinal sin. His response should be dispassionate and reasoned. He is therefore, strongly recommended not to write this letter himself, but to take advice from his MDO on what his strong or weak points are and on how to phrase his response.

Interim orders

In a significant minority of cases, the doctor will be informed in the initial complaint letter that the GMC's Case Examiners have decided to refer the matter to the Interim Orders Panel (IOP) and that there will be a hearing in a few days to decide whether interim restrictions (such as suspension) should be imposed on the doctor's registration, while the case is being investigated. The doctor will be invited to attend that hearing, which will be held in Manchester, to present his arguments as to why no order should be made.

A doctor who receives such a letter should contact his MDO without delay and arrange to see an advisor. He will also need time off work to attend the hearing.

The Interim Orders Panel has the power to restrict his ability to work when it thinks, on the basis of the complaint made, that his fitness to practise *may* be so badly impaired that he poses a risk to the public. In general, the kinds of cases referred to IOP are those where there are significant performance concerns, or where the doctor is accused of misconduct involving impropriety or a lack of probity, for example, altering medical records or presenting a false CV. Generally, the IOP will be slow to suspend a doctor when the allegations have not been tested and are unproven. They will prefer to impose conditions allowing him to continue to practise. Interim conditions will usually involve safeguards such as supervision, mentoring or restrictions on the kind of work he can do. Allegations of lack of probity are perhaps more likely to meet with an interim suspension, since no conditions are considered adequate to protect the public from a deceitful doctor.

In principle, an interim order will last for 18 months (with reviews every six months), which is the time considered sufficient for the GMC to investigate the case and, if necessary, hold a Fitness to Practise hearing.

Given the potentially serious consequences of a suspension or of conditions being imposed, it is clearly in the doctor's interests to have a good legal team representing him at the initial hearing. This should be organized by the medico-legal advisor at his MDO.

The Case Examiners

The doctor's Rule 7 response, along with the GMC's bundle of papers is then put before two Case Examiners (one medical and one lay). Their task is to consider whether on the available evidence there is a realistic prospect of establishing that his fitness to practise is impaired. If not, a number of options are available. They can close the case, issue a letter of advice, or invite him to accept a warning on his registration. In cases covering health or poor performance, they can invite him to accept certain undertakings. If however they think there is a realistic prospect of proving impaired fitness to practise, then they must refer the case to a Fitness to Practise Panel for a hearing.

Performance assessments

Complaints suggesting a pattern of poor performance may lead to a direction that the doctor's performance be assessed by a specially appointed team. His knowledge and competence will be tested objectively in various tests (knowledge tests and OSCE), and also subjectively in interviews with him and with his colleagues. A detailed report will then describe what areas of his practice are found to be acceptable, cause for concern or unacceptable. The assessors will conclude with an overall finding on whether his performance is deficient, and if so the steps they recommend to remedy those deficiencies. This report will form part of the Case Examiners' investigations and may then be the basis for either agreeing undertakings or making a referral to a Fitness to Practise Panel.

The decisions of the Case Examiners

In the majority of the cases that come before them, the Case Examiners decide not to take any further action or to simply send a letter of advice to the doctor. But they can also issue warnings or invite undertakings. The most serious cases will, however, proceed to a hearing before a Fitness to Practise Panel. In 2010, the Case Examiners' decisions were as shown in Table 3.4.

Table 3.4 Case Examiner Decisions

Refer to Panel	314
Undertakings	102
Warning	183
Advice	458
Concluded (i.e. no further action)	497
TOTAL	**1,554**

Warnings

A warning may be considered appropriate if the Case Examiners think the doctor's behaviour or performance has fallen significantly below the expected standard, but not to such a degree as to indicate impaired fitness to practise. A common example would be drink driving. A warning will remain on the doctor's registration for five years but subsequently will still remain in the public domain, albeit marked 'expired'.

In practice, the doctor might have some limited opportunity to negotiate the wording of the proposed warning. However, if this outcome is unacceptable to him, there is a right in some circumstances to challenge it before an Investigation Committee. In a significant number of cases, the Investigation Committee decides not to issue a warning after all.

Undertakings

Undertakings are a set of written agreements restricting the doctor's practice. They are likely to comprise supervision arrangements and are usually appropriate in cases concerning a doctor's health or performance. They last indefinitely, until the Case Examiners in their discretion decide that they are no longer necessary.

If undertakings are accepted then, provided that they are not confidential, they are published on the doctor's registration for as long as they are current. Even when no longer current, the inquirer will still be able to find out about them, as part of a doctor's registration history.

If the doctor does not accept the undertakings, his case will probably be referred to the Fitness to Practise Panel entailing the risk of more severe sanctions.

Referral to a Fitness to Practise Panel and erasure

The most common kinds of case referred to the Fitness to Practise Panel concern substandard treatment. In theory, a single clinical mishap should not be sufficient to establish impaired fitness to practise. What primarily concerns the GMC is a pattern of poor performance. But it does sometimes happen that a doctor with an otherwise excellent clinical reputation can find himself before a Panel because of one case that went wrong. (See the example given below.)

A Fitness to Practise Hearing is conducted in the manner of a criminal trial. At the start of the hearing, for example, the doctor is required to stand while the charges against him are read out by the Panel Secretary. Unless the hearing concerns confidential matters, such as those relating to the doctor's health, it will normally be in public. A significant difference is that since 2008 the doctor no longer has the relative protection of the criminal standard of proof, 'beyond reasonable doubt'. Now the GMC prosecutors only have to prove the case on the lesser standard of 'on the balance of probabilities' that is, the allegations are more likely to be true than not.

The hearing itself will usually take place in Manchester and will be before a Panel of at least three people (in longer cases, it should be five). Doctors in this situation are often surprised that only one member of the Panel must be a doctor, and even then, not necessarily from the same speciality.

At the end of the hearing, the Panel will decide:

1. whether (unless they are already admitted) the charges against the doctor are proven;
2. whether the charges which are admitted or found proven are sufficient to establish that his Fitness to Practise is impaired (whether by reason of misconduct, deficient performance or ill health); and
3. if so, what sanction is appropriate for the protection of the public. The sanction can range from a reprimand, to conditions, or suspension or the ultimate sanction of erasure from the register. Once erased, a doctor cannot apply to be restored to the medical register for at least five years.

Even in cases where Fitness to Practise is found not to be impaired, the Panel can be asked to consider whether to impose a warning on the doctor's registration, as an indication of its disapproval of his conduct.

It is important to appreciate that when considering whether a doctor's fitness to practise is impaired, the Panel must look not just at past failings but also at the doctor's present and future fitness to practise. A doctor who can demonstrate he understands his past failings (i.e. he has insight) and has taken action to improve his performance (i.e. remediation) may well not be impaired after all. Table 3.5 shows the outcomes of Fitness to Practise Panels in 2010.

Table 3.5 FTP Panel Outcomes

Erasure	73
Suspension	106
Conditions	37
Undertakings	5
Warning	29
Reprimand	0
Impairment – no further action	4
No impairment	65
Voluntary erasure	7
	326

A paediatric example

A Consultant Paediatrician appeared before the Fitness to Practise Panel facing allegations about his management of a sick child four years earlier. This child had the rare condition of Diamond Blackfan Anaemia. In anticipation of a bone marrow transplant, she had been prescribed Ferriprox. Five months after she began this treatment, she suffered a febrile convulsion and collapsed. She was admitted to hospital at 8 p.m., where she was looked after by a Registrar. At 3 a.m. the Registrar telephoned the consultant at his home for advice on the child's management. It was alleged that the Consultant's advice to the Registrar was not sufficiently clear and specific, particularly in relation to whether in a neutropenic patient, the antibiotics, Tazocin and Gentamicin should be administered.

The Panel weighed up the oral evidence of both the Registrar and the Consultant. It took into account variations between the Consultant's oral evidence to the Panel and his written evidence to a hospital investigation four years before, shortly after the child died. The Panel decided that he did not give clear advice to the Registrar, with the result that the antibiotics were not administered for another two to three hours.

The Panel heard evidence from a number of experts about the significance of this delay. One expert told the Panel it was reasonable to allow a breathing space in order to take stock and consider the right way forward. Another expert said that antibiotics should have been given as soon as possible after the neutropenia was documented. The Panel agreed with this view and concluded that the delay incurred by the Consultant's lack of clear instructions to the Registrar was not in the patient's best interests.

The Consultant went to see the child for himself at the hospital at 6.30 a.m. He made a written plan for her management, but it was alleged and found proved that that plan failed to provide for close monitoring by the nurses, frequent reviews by the doctors, and clinical observations every 30 minutes. The Panel referred to the fact that a shift change was due at 8 a.m. but that, having made his plan, the Consultant then left the hospital without adequately communicating it. The Panel said the Consultant should have ensured that the staff were fully aware of the seriousness of the child's condition. He should have issued a clear and emphatic plan for the frequent and close monitoring of the child's vital signs, describing what action to take if her condition deteriorated.

Having made these findings, the Panel then considered whether they amounted to misconduct and whether the Consultant's fitness to practise was impaired. They found that his acts and omissions were indeed misconduct.

However, on the question of impairment, the Consultant produced evidence of his remediation since the episode. He gave the Panel a copy of his Personal Development Plan, his CPD record, his 360° appraisal and a bundle of testimonial letters. After the events, the Consultant had approached a colleague with an interest in paediatric oncology and haematology for advice on the management of neutropenic cases. The Consultant gave evidence to the Panel that he had since reflected on the case, and that his practice in communicating with members of his team had improved. The Consultant had also used his spare time to observe practices on a Paediatric Intensive Care Unit. He told the Panel he intended to enrol on an APLS programme and a communication course.

The Panel concluded that he had taken substantial steps to remedy most of the deficiencies in his practice identified by the case. Testimonial evidence indicated he was a safe and competent practitioner. It concluded that his Fitness to Practise was not impaired.

The Panel then went on to consider whether to place a warning on the Consultant's registration. It decided *not* to do so, saying:

'The Panel has noted the circumscribed and case specific character of your misconduct. It has had regard to your creditable professional history. It has acknowledged that what happened in 2007 related to a highly unusual and specific case. It has accepted that there has been no repetition of short comings of any kind. It has taken account of the steps you have taken over remediation, and which are ongoing. It has weighed all the testimonial evidence presented on your behalf.'

The Panel said it found the Consultant to be a safe, competent and valuable practitioner of integrity, and concluded that no useful regulatory purpose would be served by imposing a warning on the doctor's registration.

The GMC in future

Two significant developments to GMC regulation are in the pipeline.

(a) Revalidation

This concept has been much discussed since the Shipman Inquiry highlighted what has been termed 'a regulatory gap' between a doctor's employer and the GMC.

> 'Some doctors [are] judged as "not bad enough" for action by the Regulator, yet not "good enough" for patients and professional colleagues in a local service to have confidence in them. There is thus a significant "regulatory gap" and it is this gap that endangers patient safety.'[6]

There were a number of public consultations on the concept of 'revalidation' as a means of closing this 'regulatory gap'. The first step towards this process was the requirement since November 2009 that to practise, a doctor must not only be registered, but must also have a licence to practise. Without that licence, it is a criminal offence to practise medicine, write prescriptions, sign death certificates or undertake any other activities which are restricted to doctors holding a licence.

In late 2012, the GMC opens the process of 'revalidation' whereby every five years a doctor's licence to practise must be renewed. To do that, the doctor must be able to demonstrate to his 'Responsible Officer' that he is up to date and remains fit to practise.

It is envisaged that every organization providing healthcare will nominate a senior practising doctor to be the GMC's Responsible Officer. He is likely to be the organization's Medical Director. He has statutory duties to the GMC and so will be the bridge crossing the gap between local clinical governance and the GMC. His duties will be to ensure that there are adequate local systems for responding to concerns about a doctor, to oversee annual appraisals for all medical staff and to make recommendations for revalidation. He will write a report on the suitability of doctors in his organization for revalidation, based on their annual appraisals over the previous five years, and on any other information drawn from clinical governance systems. Where, as a result of his submissions, the GMC's Registrar considers withdrawing a doctor's licence, the doctor will be informed and given 28 days to make representations about it. The Registrar must take those representations into account before making a decision. If he does then decide to withdraw the licence, the doctor will have the right to appeal to a Registration Appeals Panel. Equally, the GMC may well decide to put the matter through its Fitness to Practise Procedures.

What does this mean in practice for the individual doctor? He must keep a portfolio of supporting information for his annual appraisal, showing how he is keeping up to date, evaluating the quality of his work and recording feedback from colleagues and patients. The Royal Colleges for the different medical specialities will advise on the kind of material to be compiled.

The GMC has warned practitioners that appraisal discussions will be more than a mere question of collating material. 'Your appraiser will want to know what you did with the supporting information, not just that you collected it.' The doctor will be expected to reflect on how he intends to develop and modify his practice.

Discussions at appraisals may be guided by the principles of the GMC's Good Medical Practice, which have been helpfully reduced into what are called the 'Four Domains', each domain having three 'Attributes'.

The theory is that a doctor who falls short of any of the required Twelve Attributes should be picked up by the clinical governance system during the 5-year licence cycle, and given the appropriate support, so that his licence will be renewed at the end of the cycle.

The GMC says this about the closure of the 'regulatory gap':

'For the first time, employers, through Responsible Officers, will be required to make a positive statement about the Fitness to Practise of the doctors they employ. With their new responsibilities for overseeing revalidation, employers are more important than ever in promoting high standards of medical practice.'

Critics of the scheme say that a revalidation scheme based on the collection of papers and an annual appraisal will not effectively detect rogue doctors. They say that Shipman would have had his licence renewed. Critics also say that the scheme places too much power and influence in the hands of one person, the Medical Director/Responsible Officer, a feature which, they say, will draw the GMC into the politics of the workplace.

(b) Consensual disposal

Ever since the procedural reforms of 2004, the GMC, sensitive to the criticism that doctors only ever look after their own, has placed a lot of emphasis on the transparency of its procedures. Decisions about impairment and about sanction are made in public at the conclusion of a public hearing (unless the issues under consideration concern a doctor's health in which case the hearing is in private). This is intended to maintain public confidence in the profession.

However, what has tended to happen is that after several days of exhausting and stressful evidence, although facts may have been proven against the doctor, it turns out that he can show insight and remediation. His Fitness to Practise may have been impaired at the time, but it is now no longer impaired. In that case, there is no finding of impairment and the worst that can happen is a warning. The paediatric example given above is a case in question. Was the hearing worth it?

Add to that the rising number of complaints, the rising number of hearings every year and the rising cost, and we find that the GMC is now thinking about dealing with at least some of its cases in a different way. The phrase 'consensual disposal' has been coined for the suggestion that the GMC and the doctor engage in some discussion about agreeing a sanction without the need for a hearing or witnesses. But would this kind of process undermine public confidence and create a perception of deals done 'behind closed doors'?

A recent consultation showed a large measure of support for the idea in principle. It was thought it might be most suitable for cases where there were no significant disputes about the facts. But it was also considered that there would be some cases in which such a process would be inappropriate, although it was difficult to establish what kind of cases these might be. More detailed proposals on the idea are now being developed by the GMC.

8   The role of the doctor

It is a term of all NHS employment contracts that staff must assist with investigations. Likewise, it is a professional requirement of the GMC's Good Medical Practice. A doctor who is asked to provide a written statement of events as part of any investigation– whether an internal hospital inquiry or a Coroner's inquiry must cooperate. Equally, he must be very conscious that what he writes now may be referred to in later proceedings. He therefore needs to be accurate. If there is any risk of trouble in the future, a doctor would be well advised to contact his MDO and ask for his proposed statement to be looked over by a medico-legal adviser.

Witness statements

A doctor who is asked to prepare a witness statement concerning the care of a patient should always be provided with a copy of the relevant set of patient records to assist him.

Although a witness statement should be prepared as soon as possible after the event, so that the details are fresh in the mind, the doctor should not allow himself to be rushed. Accuracy is more important.

Here are some tips on writing a well laid out and clear witness statement:

Formal requirements
- Write on one side of the paper only.
- Type the statement and bind it using one staple in the top left-hand coroner. Have a decent left and right margin and double space the document.
- Use a heading to orientate the reader for example 'Statement of Bob Smith following the death of Augustus Clark on E Ward at Pilkington Hospital on 22 November 2006'.
- Number the pages and identify the statement in the top right-hand corner of each page for example 'Page 2 Witness Statement of Bob SMITH'.

- Number paragraphs and appendices.
- Refer to documents and names in capitals and express numbers as figures.
- Attach copies of protocols or other documents referred to for example staff rota or clinical observations chart.
- Sign and date it.
- End with a statement of truth: 'I believe that the contents of this statement are true.'
- Spellcheck the statement.

Content
- Before starting, decide 'What are the issues?'
- Write a chronology. This will provide the structure.
- In the first paragraph, witnesses should set out who they are, their occupation and where they work (currently and at the time of the incident). It is important to orientate the reader, so a short CV is helpful. In more complex cases a fuller CV can be appended
- There should be a main heading and subheadings.
- Use short sentences (a sentence that goes on for more than 2 lines may be too long) and paragraphs (aim for about 3 sentences per paragraph).
- Do not stray into another witness's evidence.
- Statements should contain no retrospective opinions, only contemporaneous opinions. Avoid statements like, 'I thought for years this was going to happen.' Contemporaneous opinions should be backed up by facts. So, when stating a professional opinion, for example a diagnosis, explain the thinking behind the opinion
- Do not use jargon. If technical terms have to be used, consider the use of a glossary and/or diagrams. Try to make the statement accessible to a nonclinician.
- Avoid pseudo-legal language such as 'I was proceeding in a northerly direction . . .'
- Identify individuals as they are introduced to the narrative.
- Ambiguous expressions such as 'I would have done such and such' should be avoided. If the doctor does not recall what he did, he should say so clearly. If, based on his normal practice, he believes he did such and such, then this should be made clear too.

Presenting oral evidence

Having looked at negligence claims, disciplinary hearings, Coroner's hearings and GMC hearings, it is appropriate to say a few words about how to give evidence. For the way a witness presents his evidence affects the weight given to it by the Court/Inquiry/Tribunal.

Remember that a witness's role is to assist the Tribunal. He is not there to argue with the barrister.

The barristers may try to draw witnesses into an argument. They may also use other techniques to disconcert them, such as moving between multiple documents. Once the witness recognizes that they are just techniques, they can watch out for them and so remain in control.

The lawyer is only doing his job. Witnesses have to separate themselves from the evidence and not get angry.

Before giving evidence, witnesses should:

- reread and think about all the evidence including the records, protocols, national guidelines and professional standards;
- reread witness statements and Court/Inquiry documents (if appropriate) and ask their lawyer to explain anything they do not understand;
- check with the lawyers whether there are any other documents they would like the witness to read, such as clinical studies;
- tell the lawyers about any mistakes or omissions in the witness statement;
- visit the courtroom beforehand; ask the Court for a tour;
- if possible see the Court/Inquiry 'in action' beforehand;
- plan the route to the hearing, arrange where to meet everyone and work out what to wear;
- exchange telephone numbers with the legal team;
- put the Court telephone number into their mobile phone;
- practise taking the oath and giving their credentials.

At the hearing

- report to the reception desk where you will need to register;
- be prepared to come into contact with family members and media representatives;
- keep conversations to a minimum and nonverbal communications appropriate;
- on entering the courtroom sit down and do not talk;
- stand up when the Judge/Panel arrives and then be seated;
- the proceedings will be recorded; be prepared to speak clearly and slowly;
- pause before answering any questions;
- listen carefully to the question;
- deliver your answers to the Judge/Panel; the best way to ensure this is to stand with your feet facing the Judge/Panel and turn from the hips to take questions from the lawyers;
- try to keep answers to questions brief and to the point;
- try to eliminate passion from your answers.

No-one, not even a seasoned expert witness enjoys the stress of giving evidence. But to do so is part of a doctor's professional duty.

9 Emotional repercussions

Many doctors take criticism extremely personally, even if the complaint is relatively straightforward and can be put to rest without too much difficulty. Each doctor will react differently. The experience may leave him feeling

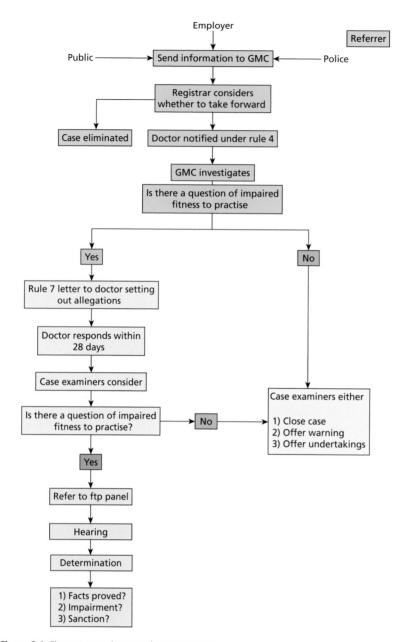

Figure 3.1 Fitness to practice procedure: a summary.

scarred. Some may find that the complaint takes a physical toll on them. Some may even leave the profession altogether. Others seem able to take a relaxed attitude, at least on the surface.

Stress associated with complaints can lead to anxiety, depression and on rare occasions even suicide. It can impinge on the doctor's work and family life. People deal with stress in different ways, but talking to colleagues, friends and family can help. The solicitor and the medico-legal advisor at a doctor's MDO are on hand to help and to listen to concerns. They are there to provide emotional support as much as legal advice.

The GMC has produced a useful leaflet, available on line, called, 'Your Health Matters' providing doctors with advice about looking after their own health. It lists numerous sources of support for doctors experiencing stress or depression.

The British Medical Association also offers a 24-hour counselling service with the opportunity to talk to a counsellor or a doctor on 08459 200 169. A doctor may need the help of a GP, psychotherapist or psychiatrist. Some Deaneries, such as the London Deanery, offer free emotional support and psychotherapy to doctors suffering from stress or emotional ill health. Doctors can self-refer to this service. In London the service (called MedNet) is run by Consultant Psychiatrists (020 8938 2411). So there are many sources of help for the doctor suffering from stress or anxiety.

10   Conclusion

We hope that this final part of the book has clarified the procedures which may take place after a medical error.

The reader may well be daunted by the number and complexity of the investigations which can be made. However he should take heart. Although dealing with a complaint may be *very* stressful there is always high quality professional help available. Our advice is to make full use of it.

The other point to make is that error is part of the human condition. In 2010 there were 7100 complaints to the GMC and it is thus not uncommon for a doctor to be referred. Fortunately, only a small proportion concern paediatricians. All doctors make mistakes, even excellent ones and even those who sit on GMC Fitness to Practise Panels. Doctors who make mistakes may become better at their jobs as a result, and can go on to have successful and productive careers. So never lose heart, but do reflect on errors and pay heed to any lessons that can be learnt.

References and further reading

1. Patient trigger tool. www.institute.nhs.uk/safercare/paediatric_safer_care/the_paediatric_trigger_tool.html
2. G Scally, LJ Donaldson (1998) Clinical Governance and the drive for quality improvement in the new NHS in England. *BMJ* 317: 61–5.
3. The Citizen's Charter: Raising the Standard, Cm 1599, (1991) http://www.parliament.uk/briefing-papers/RP95-66.pdf
4. The Local Authorities Social Services and NHS Complaints (England) Regulations (2009) http://www.legislation.gov.uk/uksi/2009/309/regulation/2/made

5. Royal College of Paediatricians and Child Health (2008) Guidance on Child Death Review Processes.
6. Department of Health (2006) Good Doctors, Safer Patients: Proposals to strengthen the system to assure and improve the performance of doctors and to protect the safety of patients. http://www.dh.gov.uk/en/ Publicationsandstatistics/Publications/PublicationsPolicyAndGuidance/ DH_4137232

Index

Avoiding Errors in Paediatrics, First Edition. Joseph E. Raine, Kate Williams and Jonathan Bonser.
© 2013 John Wiley & Sons, Ltd. Published 2013 by Blackwell Publishing Ltd.